E/28979   €10.95.
616.083 DIN   x

WITHDRAWN

D0275710

AN INTRODUCTION TO
THE SOCIAL HISTORY OF NURSING

AN INTRODUCTION TO
THE SOCIAL HISTORY OF
NURSING

ROBERT DINGWALL,
ANNE MARIE RAFFERTY
AND CHARLES WEBSTER

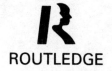

ROUTLEDGE

First published in 1988 by Routledge
a division of Routledge, Chapman and Hall
11 New Fetter Lane, London EC4P 4EE

© 1988 Robert Dingwall, Anne Marie Rafferty and Charles Webster

Printed in Great Britain by Billing & Sons Ltd, Worcester

All rights reserved. No part of this book may be
reprinted or reproduced or utilized in any form or
by any electronic, mechanical, or other means, now
known or hereafter invented, including photocopying
and recording, or in any information storage or
retrieval system, without permission in writing from
the publishers.

British Library Cataloguing in Publication Data

Dingwall, Robert
    An introduction to the social history of nursing.
    1. Great Britain. Medicine. Nursing, to 1979
    I. Title II. Rafferty, Anne Marie III. Webster, Charles, *1936–*
    610.73'0941

    ISBN 0–415–01785–8 Hbk
    ISBN 0–415–01786–6 Pbk

Contents

Acknowledgements

A book like this necessarily draws on the work of many colleagues whose hard labour on primary sources has provided the foundation on which we could build. We would like to thank a number of friends and associates in Oxford and elsewhere who have not only commented on drafts but also contributed generously from their own unpublished researches. Among them we should particularly mention Kate Robinson, who prompted the whole project, Irvine Loudon, Elizabeth Peretz, Alastair Gray, Phil Strong, Malcolm Colledge, Peter Bartrip, Miranda Mugford, John Keown, Celia Davies, Mick Carpenter, Pat Hearn, and Renata Langford. We would particularly like to thank Anne Summers for advance reference to her book *Angels and Citizens: British Women as Military Nurses 1854–1914* (Summers 1988). We would also like to thank Margaret Lynch and Anne Wiles for their consumers' reactions to early drafts, and Linda Peterson and Jeanette Price who typed the manuscript.

The preparation of this book was supported by a contract from the Distance Learning Centre at South Bank Polytechnic.

Glossary of abbreviations

AWA	Association of Workers in Asylums
BMA	British Medical Association
C(E) THV	Council for the (Education and) Training of Health Visitors
CMB	Central Midwives Board
COHSE	Confederation of Health Service Employees
COS	Charity Organisation Society
DHSS	Department of Health and Social Security
GNC	General Nursing Council
HMC	Hospital Management Committee
LCC	London County Council
LGB	Local Government Board
NALGO	National Association of Local Government Officers
NAWU	National Asylum Workers Union
NHS	National Health Service
NHSTA	National Health Service Training Authority
NSPCC	National Society for the Prevention of Cruelty to Children
ODA	Operating Department Assistant
RCM	Royal College of Midwives
RCN	Royal College of Nursing
RCOG	Royal College of Obstetricians and Gynaecologists
RHB	Royal Hospital Board
RMN	Registered Mental Nurse
(R)MPA	(Royal) Medico-Psychological Association
RSI	Royal Sanitary Institute
RSPCA	Royal Society for the Prevention of Cruelty to Animals
SEN	State Enrolled Nurse
SRN	State Registered Nurse
TUC	Trades Union Congress
UKCC	United Kingdom Central Council for Nursing, Midwifery and Health Visiting
VAD	Voluntary Aid Detachment
WSIA	Women Sanitary Inspectors' Association

Chapter one

Nurses and Servants

If you could travel backwards in time to 1800, what would the health care system look like? The first thing to grasp is that it would not look like a system at all. Since 1948, most of us have grown up with a pretty clear idea of what a hospital is, what a doctor is, what a nurse is, and so on. In our lifetime there has been a fair degree of consensus about what is and is not valid and reliable medical knowledge. If you looked at health care in 1800, you would find that none of these assumptions hold true. There was no generally accepted body of medical knowledge so that rival theories circulated freely and competitively. There was no legal definition of a doctor and few restrictions on the practice of healing. The Royal Colleges of Physicians and Surgeons and the Society of Apothecaries all competed to licence suppliers of medical treatment and to protect the privileges of those whom they had admitted. However, they would only have served relatively well-off people living in or near major towns. Elsewhere, medical care would be given by family members, especially women, using treatments handed down in the local community or taken from books of home remedies, or by anybody from the neighbourhood who could build up some reputation as a healer, a bonesetter, a herbalist, or a midwife. These might be ordinary villagers or people with some education like a parson or a squire, or their wives. Even among the elite physicians, only the most successful healers could work full-time and make a living at this trade (Waddington 1985: 180–90).

Architecturally, the voluntary hospitals might have looked more familiar, but, of course, some of their buildings are still in use. Wards were large, rectangular rooms holding between fifteen and thirty patients in parallel rows of beds on each side. If you were to examine the patients, however, you might wonder how many of them were sufficiently ill to justify their place. People seldom died

1

in the voluntary hospitals – death rates were probably no more than 10 per cent of admissions (Woodward 1974: 123–42). This was achieved largely by refusing admission to people who appeared to be seriously ill or infectious. The typical patient would be more likely to be suffering some sort of minor surgical problem – a fracture, a skin ulcer, a fistula, or a boil. As a result, the whole atmosphere would have been more reminiscent of some kind of convalescent home. At the Royal Devon and Exeter Hospital, for example, patients were allowed to come and go as they pleased in the daytime until the 1830s, provided they did not return drunk. They were expected to help with the domestic chores, feeding the pigs, pumping water and serving meals (Hawker 1987).

To understand why patients were selected in this fashion, we must look at the way these hospitals were financed. Although there were some older institutions, like St Thomas's and St Bartholomew's Hospitals in London, which had substantial incomes from endowments, most of the newer foundations depended upon current subscriptions from well-off members of the community. Thus, it was not in the hospital's interest that it acquired the reputation of being a place which killed people. Moreover, subscribers expected something in return for their donations. This might be preferential treatment in contracts to supply the hospital, for example, but more generally it was the right to nominate patients for a stay of six to eight weeks. These nominations would be considered at a weekly meeting of the governors which would then decide who was to be admitted, a policy that also tended to exclude acute patients.

Despite this charitable basis, the patients were no more likely to be very poor than they were to be very sick. Although the middle and upper classes made little use of any type of hospital until the twentieth century, voluntary hospital patients were likely to need sufficient resources or sponsorship to provide a deposit or guarantee against possible funeral expenses. In addition, there was often some admission charge. At Guy's Hospital, London, patients in 1788 were expected to arrive

> with a change of Body-Linen, Stockings, Neckcloth, Stock and Handkerchief, and to pay to the Sister Two Shillings and Ninepence for two Towels, a Tin pot, a Knife, a Spoon, an Earthen Plate and five Pairs of Sheets. (H.C. Cameron 1954 *Mr. Guy's Hospital 1726–1948*. Quoted by Abel-Smith 1964: 10)

Except for patients with venereal infections, however, actual subsistence and treatment would be free. Unfortunately, we know very little about who the patients were. Governors' minute books record discussions of the eligibility of domestic servants or apprentices of the subscribers, which may give us some clues. The issue there was whether an employer should pay for their care directly or whether the employer's subscription should cover their hospital treatment. Given the importance of personal recommendation, though, it seems reasonable to suppose that most patients would have had some such connection, if not directly, then through friends or family members. Even so, there were not very many of them. In 1800, there were about 4,000 hospital beds in England and Wales, of which about 3,000 would have been occupied at any one time. That was one bed for every 5,000 persons (Abel-Smith 1964: 1).

What happened to everyone else? The answer seems to be that they remained in their own homes with the benefit of such medical attendance as they could afford and considered appropriate. Those who needed treatment and were unable to pay for it had to rely on the provisions of the Poor Law. This is the collective name for a series of acts of parliament dating back to Elizabeth I which required parish officers to levy property taxes to provide for orphans, the old, the mentally disordered, the unemployed, and the sick. This help took two forms: 'outdoor' relief which described services or money furnished to people in their homes and 'indoor' relief which would involve the person's removal to a workhouse. In fact, there were relatively few workhouses built before 1834 so that most relief was provided on an outdoor basis (Henriques 1979: 17–19).

Poor Law medical practice at this time has been depicted as a service provided by quacks or underpaid parish surgeons who were either so overloaded or so incompetent as to deny paupers adequate treatment, by the standards of the day (Hodgkinson 1967: 8–9). More recently, however, Loudon (1987: 228–48) has shown that this office was relatively prestigious and well-rewarded, with its holders being reimbursed on the basis of their private fees for each item of treatment. The competition to hold such posts was reflected in the high quality of care offered to acute cases. It is true that there was no legal restriction on who could be appointed as a parish surgeon until the 1860s, following the creation of the Medical Register and the statutory definition of the medical profession. But, as Loudon points out, the rapid mobilization of medical officers during the 1831–2 cholera epidemic certainly suggests that the parishes had a clear perception of who was and was not a competent practitioner, even in the absence of national standards. The negative picture may represent an over-reliance on writings by critics of the Poor Law as part of their campaign for

3

change, although, as Loudon concedes, there is some evidence that the more restrictive attitudes which inspired the 1834 reform of the Poor Law (see pp. 11 and 30) were already leading to a deterioration in the service during the 1820s.

Nurses before nursing

This sketch of health care at the beginning of the nineteenth century will serve as a background for our discussion of the development of general nursing. The first difficulty we face, however, is in defining what counts as nursing so that we know what to include in our analysis. In the early nineteenth century nursing was not an identifiable and self-conscious occupation. Anybody could freely describe themselves as 'a nurse' and call what they did 'nursing' until the General Nursing Council Register became operational in 1923. Even since then it has continued to be difficult to draw a boundary between nursing and non-nursing work and to discriminate between those parts which are reserved for members of the occupation, those which are shared by members of other occupations, and those which may be done by anybody. Thus it is important to find a way of differentiating between 'nursing work' and 'work done by nurses'.

The relationship between work and occupations is a topic which has long been of interest to sociologists. However, the main application of this interest to nursing has previously been confined to the question of whether it is or is not a profession. Although we shall not be pursuing that issue here, its prevalence obliges us to explain our decision.

The question about the status of nursing is particularly associated with what is known as the trait or attribute approach to the study of professions. This involves drawing up a list of criteria against which various occupations can be matched (e.g. Greenwood 1957). Those meeting all or most are accepted as professions, those meeting some criteria are often called semi-professions and those which meet few or none are ruled out of the category. This approach has, however, been effectively discredited by Millerson (1964) and Roth (1974) who have shown how vague and inconsistent these lists are and how they tend to be compiled to yield particular results. Moreover, this kind of classification ends up with very little positive to say about either the organization of work or the organization of society. It is largely a matter of ranking occupations on some sort of prestige scale. One way round this problem which was explored by some writers was a proposal to study professionalization as if it were an evolutionary process by which certain occupations enhanced their status (e.g. Caplow 1954, Wilensky 1964). But this also foundered on the problem of producing a usable definition of what a profession was, as the end-state of that process (Turner and Hodge 1970: 23, Johnson 1972: 31).

As Becker (1970) has pointed out, the fundamental problem is that the word 'profession' is used for two incompatible purposes. One is as a 'folk concept', a way in which anyone can describe a particular occupation or activity with respect: hence the 'professional foul' in soccer, for example (cf. Horobin 1983: 84–95). In this sense it is a badge of honour which is tied to particular societies in a particular historical period (Freidson 1983: 23–6). The other use is as a label for a group of occupations which form a meaningful unit for sociological analysis.

Various attempts were made during the 1970s to develop this latter approach. Freidson (1970a) suggested that the term should be defined in relation to occupations which had achieved 'functional autonomy', the ability to determine their own conditions of work, although he has subsequently rejected attempts to treat this as if it were an attribute and identify it with self-employment (Freidson 1986: 123–5). Johnson (1972, 1977, 1982) has explored the ways in which professions could be delineated as occupations which stand in a particular relationship to the political structure of Western societies, while Larson (1977) has treated them as occupations which have established a distinctive measure of control over the market for their services.[1] Freidson (1986) has attempted to unite these lines of analysis by proposing that professions are inter-mediaries between bodies of formal knowledge and the human activities which apply them. This role is both a source of autonomy and a basis for economic, legal and political privilege.

While many of these ideas can be usefully employed in the analysis of nursing, their direct relevance is limited, as Freidson (1970b: 20–2) observes, by the position of the occupation in a medically dominated division of labour. It therefore seems more helpful to start from the fundamental questions identified by Hughes (1971: 283–417) and pursued in various ways by Freidson (1978), Dingwall (1983a, 1983b), and Abbott (1986). This would absorb the study of professions into a more general sociology of occupations. Rather than asking 'What is a profession?', we should be asking 'What kinds of occupation are there and how do they divide the work that has to be done in a society?' The division of the workforce into occupations creates a scheme for the social classification of work. There is no necessary relationship between the categories of this scheme, occupations, and the array of tasks that need to be done in a society. So we can ask why that array is carved up in one way or another at different times and in different places.

We can draw an analogy between the social organization of work and the development of a city. Think of all the work that has to be done in a society as the land on which the city is built. Now think of all the different occupations you can name as the buildings put on that land. But cities are not static. Their boundaries change. Redevelopment is occurring all the time. Some buildings are being improved and enlarged. Sometimes plots will be cleared and new constructions put up on them. In the same way, the definition of work is something which may change over time. New occupations may be created, like computer programmers in the 1950s. Others may disappear, like ostlers when the stage coach gave way to the steam train. Some occupations divide as surgeons did from barbers in the sixteenth century. Others fuse, as physicians, surgeons and apothecaries did in the mid-Victorian period.

One way of viewing the Nurses Registration Act 1919 is as a licence for a prominent group of people to redevelop an area of the city. But the possible form of the building they erected was partly determined by the nature of the site and the previous attempts to develop it. Some of these were incorporated in the new scheme and others excluded. A number were subsequently annexed, a move which was recognized finally by the Nurses, Midwives and Health Visitors Act 1979. This book is rather like an archaeological dig that attempts to trace the earlier foundations which run across the site and may divide it in a very different fashion.

It seems logical, then, to begin from the core activity of providing direct care for sick people and to trace the changes in its ownership and its association with other tasks such as the delivery of babies and the prevention or management of health-related problems.[2] What did the care of the sick consist of in the early nineteenth century and who gave it?

Then, as now, the greatest part of the care required by the sick involved some kind of assistance with activities of daily living that they were unable to carry out for themselves. Indeed, before the introduction of modern techniques of diagnosis, this would have been the main way of defining someone as ill, that they were involuntarily unable to look after their own bodily needs. Care at this level involves basic assistance with feeding, toileting or personal hygiene. At its margins this form of care would merge into two other types of involvement. One would be the simple techniques of pre-industrial medicine – diet, dressings, poultices, herbal infusions, etc. – and the other would be the spiritual care of the terminally sick or injured.

If we go back to the first half of the nineteenth century with this broad description of nursing care, we can identify four categories of people who are involved in its provision. The first, and almost certainly the largest, would have been members of the sick person's household caring for them at home. Their informal work might have been assisted by one or other of two types of paid helper, which we shall describe as the 'handywoman' and the 'private nurse'. Both of these groups were independent, self-employed workers and they can be distinguished mainly by whether they were providing a cheap service for the poor or a premium service for the better-off. Because their services were being traded, they can reasonably be regarded as part of the official workforce, although neither occupation is well-defined and the handywomen, in particular, may also have been involved in criminal work. There was some movement between domestic and institutional employment and the hospitals show a similar social division among their staff. We shall, then, organize our analysis around the work and the workers rather than their particular location. Almost all of these informal or official carers would have been women.

The fourth category of workers were all men. They were types of medical attendant – 'apothecaries', 'dressers', 'residents', 'clinical clerks' – whose memory is preserved only by job titles for junior staff in some rather traditional hospitals. Originally, these men would have been the subordinates or apprentices of more powerful or prestigious practitioners. They were the people who actually administered such routine treatments as were used in hospitals before the nineteenth century. Outside the hospital many of those same treatments would have been given by the other types of carer, either as directed by an adviser, who might or might not be a medical practitioner, or following traditional ideas, passed on by word of mouth or in books of home remedies.

Domestic nursing

It would now be impossible to quantify the division of nursing work between informal and official carers in pre-industrial England. On the basis of the surviving diaries and literary sources, however, it seems reasonable to infer that most care would have been given on a relatively informal basis by other members of the sick person's household.

We would emphasize the contribution of the household rather than the family. There is a romantic view of the past which supposes that people tended to live from one generation to the next in the same house or neighbourhood in large and inter-related families. This gave communities a capacity to care for the sick which they are unable or unwilling to provide in our own time.

In fact, families of this type were relatively uncommon in England. Over the period 1622–1854, only 6 per cent of households contained three generations of kin: over 70 per cent consisted of two generations alone (Laslett 1983: 98). Several factors are involved in this. First, the potential demands for care were more limited than in the twentieth century. For example, between 1539 and 1843, the proportion of the population over 60 never exceeded 9.7 per cent, compared with 21 per cent in 1985 (Laslett 1983: 111, Central Statistical Office 1987: Table 2.4). Second, the number of potential carers and the extent of their obligations was limited by the relatively small size of families and the high rate of marriages broken by death. Although an average woman was likely to have just under seven children, of whom three-quarters would survive infancy, the typical marriage only produced just over four. Between one-third and one-half of all children lost one or both parents during their childhood, creating complex two-generation households of single parent families and families of orphans being brought up by remarried step parents (Hair 1982, Laslett 1983: 113–19). Finally, even where carers were theoretically available, they were quite likely to have moved out of the locality. From the sixteenth century, and before, there is evidence of considerable population mobility (Clark 1979, Laslett 1983: 75).

It is probably more important, then, to recognize the role of household servants. Although grand establishments were rare, most households were likely to contain one or more servants at some time or other (Laslett 1983: 12–16). The household was an economic as well as a social unit. Its land, craft or trade could absorb a certain amount of labour for maximum productivity. But the human resources of a family fluctuate. Before children are born, both spouses may be fully available for work. When children are small, labour must be diverted to their care and a shortage may arise. Conversely, as the children grow up, their labour may become surplus and the household resources insufficient to support them (cf. Goody 1958). Domestic service, for both men and women, was a way of smoothing out these variations, with servants being imported and children being exported to match the supply and demand for labour in different households.

But when a household was affected by the sickness or incapacity of one of its members, some decision would have to be made about whether it was more efficient to deal with this by diverting some existing resources into caring for that person or by engaging an additional servant. Where the ordinary servants' work was fairly specialized or the incapacity fairly predictable, as with childbirth and postpartum care, it seems plausible to suppose that it would be judged more efficient to import extra help than to divert others from productive activities. Where there were no other servants, hiring one to care for the sick person might enable a spouse to continue to generate some income.

While this is essentially a speculative application of simple economic theory, it does have the merit of accounting for the evidence of considerable numbers of casually employed nurses. Before looking at these, it is perhaps worth underlining that the caring capacity of the community in pre-industrial England reflects a society in which servants were much more common than they are today. As such it cannot be a basis for simple comparisons between then and now.

The handywomen

As Abel-Smith (1960) pointed out, the provision of nursing care by village women, and, we might add, by working-class women in towns or cities, has been largely ignored by historians of the occupation. The position has not changed greatly since so that any account inevitably depends upon scraps of information in the margins of other studies, although, in fairness, the lack of documentation would make it hard to write a full historical treatment. Nevertheless, 'handywomen' were probably the largest group of paid carers operating throughout the nineteenth century and well into the twentieth.

Much of the conventional image of the handywomen is formed by fictional accounts, which can be treated as evidence of characters whom readers were expected to recognize from life. Perhaps the most celebrated is Sarah Gamp, from Charles Dickens's 1844 novel, *Martin Chuzzlewit*. This is how we first meet her:

> Mr. Pecksniff had been to the undertaker and was now upon his way to another office in the train of mourning: a female functionary, a nurse and watcher, and performer of nameless offices about the persons of the dead. . . . This lady lodged at a bird fancier's, next door but one to the celebrated mutton-pie

shop, and directly opposite to the original cat's meat warehouse.
. . . It was a little house, and this was the more convenient; for
Mrs. Gamp, being, in her highest walk of art, a monthly nurse,
or, as her sign-board boldly had it, 'Midwife', and lodging in the
first-floor front, was easily assailable at night . . .

She was a fat old woman, this Mrs. Gamp, with a husky voice
and a moist eye, which she had a remarkable power of turning
up, and only showing the white of it. Having very little neck, it
cost her some trouble to look over herself, if one may say so, at
those to whom she talked. She wore a very rusty black gown,
rather the worse for snuff, and a shawl and bonnet to
correspond. In these dilapidated articles of dress she had, on
principle, arrayed herself, time out of mind, on such occasions
as the present; for this at once expressed a decent amount of
veneration for the deceased, and invited the next of kin to
present her with a fresher suit of weeds: an appeal so frequently
successful, that the very fetch and ghost of Mrs. Gamp, bonnet
and all, might be seen hanging up, any hour of the day, in at
least a dozen of the second-hand clothes shops about Holborn.
The face of Mrs. Gamp – the nose in particular – was somewhat
red and swollen, and it was difficult to enjoy her society without
becoming conscious of a smell of spirits. Like most persons who
have attained a great eminence in their profession, she took
hers very kindly; insomuch that, setting aside her natural
predilections as a woman, she went to a lying-in or a laying-out
with equal zest and relish.

Mrs. Gamp is an independent practitioner but Dickens also
depicts her hospital counterpart in Betsy Prig 'recommended from
(St) Bartholomew's'.

These descriptions are, of course, contrived by their authors to
achieve particular objectives. In evaluating them as accounts of
early nineteenth century nursing, we must consider what those
objectives were and how they shape the characters depicted in
them with comparison with other surviving data. Charles Dickens's
novels almost invariably carry some message about the social ills of
early nineteenth century England. As Abel-Smith (1960: 5)
observed, it is still not unusual for reformers to overstate the evils
they hope to correct.

Nevertheless, it is clear that such accounts can be accepted as
accurate in certain respects. Firstly, nursing at this level was a very
basic form of domestic service. The following descriptions are
from St Thomas's and Guy's Hospitals, respectively, in the 1850s.

As regards the nurses or ward-maids, these are much in the

condition of housemaids and require little teaching beyond that of poultice-making which is easily acquired, and the enforcement of cleanliness and attention to patients' wants. They need not be of the class of people required for sisters, not having such responsibility . . . (South 1857)

For the more subordinate appointment of nurse, which at the time referred to included not only attendance on the more immediate wants of the sick but the cleaning and scrubbing of ward floors and of the staircases of the hospital, it was necessary to select from a class of inferior grade to the others . . . preference is given to a good class of domestic servants between the age of 20 and 40 years. After a woman has taken to the work it rarely happens that she leaves it. (Steele 1874)

But it does not necessarily follow from this that patients were badly treated. A hundred years earlier, the 1752 regulations of the Manchester Infirmary had run together these two types of work but emphasized their common duties in requiring 'That the Nurses and Servants obey the Matron as their Mistress and that they behave with Tenderness to the Patients, and Civility and Respect to Strangers'. Early in the nineteenth century, the matron of the Radcliffe Infirmary in Oxford would simply advertise for a 'careful woman' or promote one of the existing servants if a nurse were required. Part of the attraction of the work seems to have been the acquisition of skills which would be useful in seeking positions in private households upon marriage. The Salisbury Infirmary in 1796 advertised the value of nursing to 'young respectable women who would be taught how to look after sick people' (Abel-Smith 1960: 4–7, Woodward 1974: 24–35). Whatever the realities of the situation, statements like these do indicate at least an aspiration to create a caring environment. The extent to which this was achieved in practice is underlined by the independent report of the Charity Commissioners on St Thomas's Hospital in 1836 which documents a disciplined and responsible system (Rivett 1986: 36–7).

Conditions were undeniably more problematic under the Poor Law which was coming to provide most of the institutional care of the sick (Abel-Smith 1960: 4). The system had been completely reformed in 1834 with the object of restricting outdoor relief. There is a considerable historical controversy about these changes but, very crudely, it seems that the Poor Law had been exploited by farmers to pay low wages to workers whose income was then made up from the poor rate. This had increased costs and thrown an unfair burden on other ratepayers. The Poor Law Amendment

Act 1834 attacked this problem by imposing penalties on labourers who sought assistance in the expectation that this would be transmitted back to the farmers in demands for full wages. The main penalty was removal to the workhouse where the conditions were to be designed to be worse than those of the poorest employed person, what was called the 'principle of less eligibility'. It was not originally intended that this should be applied to the sick and the aged, who should either receive outdoor relief or be accommodated in 'distinct, quiet and comfortable abodes'. In practice, however, there were strong pressures and incentives for both groups to be removed into the general workhouse where they received the same treatment as the able-bodied unemployed (Henriques 1979: 26–65).

The workhouses gradually filled up with the chronic sick and the elderly. As the able-bodied migrated to the towns in search of work these were the people who were left in the rural areas with no other potential carers. When periods of prosperity drew the able-bodied into work, especially in 1844–6, their places were taken by longer-stay inmates so that, when the economy turned down again, there was simply no room in the workhouse and outdoor relief had to be reinstituted for the unemployed. The spirit of less eligibility continued to rule, however, in the clothing, diet and regime of the workhouse.

Most of the direct care was provided by other pauper inmates. This was preferred because it was a form of work that did not compete with outside trades, it was unpleasant enough to discourage people from staying in the workhouse for longer than necessary and it was cheap, since the pauper nurses did not have to be paid market wages. They simply received extra privileges in the form of food or liquor or token cash payments. At the Strand workhouse in the 1860s, for instance, pauper nurses were given a glass of gin 'for laying out the dead and other specially repulsive duties'. As a result able-bodied nurses left as soon as they could get other employment and the burden of care fell on the least infirm of those who remained. Pauper nurses tended to be elderly women with little prospect of employment outside the workhouse, except when the guardians allowed them out to nurse poor people receiving outdoor relief (Crowther 1981: 227). At the Strand, 14 out of 18 pauper nurses were over 60 and 4 were over 70. Only 8 could read the labels on the medicines. Two trembled and coughed all day and were too frail to lift any patient. But it is also clear that some workhouses did manage to make the system work. The *Lancet* commission, whose report was a key text for reformers in the 1860s, singled out the pauper nurses in Islington as 'well-conducted, zealous and well managed' (Abel-Smith 1960: 10–14, Hodgkinson 1967: 488–9).

Both before and after 1834, however, a good deal of nursing care was provided as outdoor relief. This included both midwifery and assistance with sickness (Stocks 1960: 92–3, Donnison 1977: 59, Smith 1979: 41–55, Hodgkinson 1967: 285, Baly 1987: 2). The picture which emerges is one of relatively poor women, perhaps widows or deserted wives, providing a service to other poor people. Their payments from the Poor Law might well have functioned, in effect, as a form of outdoor relief for themselves. Sometimes they would work for paupers, sometimes for people who were simply poor but not so impoverished as to qualify for relief. Again, though, there are hints of a concern for standards which belies the simple chronicle of abuse. Acland's memoirs of the 1854 cholera outbreak in Oxford record that the Poor Law guardians kept a list of 'respectable women' who were willing to do home nursing. Patients could either hire nurses from this list or be nursed by one of them at the guardians' expense (Dean and Bolton 1980: 93). The existence of such lists presupposes criteria of respectability and a desire to encourage it.

Although we have questioned the suggestion that Sarah Gamp's character is typical of handywoman nurses, her duties probably were: nursing the sick, delivering babies, and laying out the dead. To these one might well add procuring abortions and disposing of unwanted infants (Smith 1979: 67–80, Keown 1988). Out of these various tasks, some handywomen might have developed a particular reputation as counsellors on the health problems of women and children, which were of little interest to doctors in general until the twentieth century. Not all handywomen would necessarily have taken on all these tasks and it is doubtful whether more than a few made a full-time living from them. It may be better to see nursing as an interlude in their work as cleaners or laundresses.

The handywomen had no consciousness of themselves as an occupational group: indeed this is one of the reasons why so little documentary evidence is readily available. They simply filled a traditional social and economic role in their locality. This was an important factor in their survival in community-based work. As we show later, handywomen remained serious competitors to certified midwives and district nurses until the 1930s and 1940s.

Private nurses

If the handywoman was part of the traditional organization of care among the poor, the private duty nurse was equally well-established among the middle and upper classes. However, whereas the handywoman was working essentially with clients of her own class, the private duty nurse was a servant of her social superiors. Jane Austen describes one such woman, Nurse Rooke, in *Persuasion* (1818).

(Mrs Smith) could not call herself an invalid now compared with her state on first reaching Bath. Then, she had indeed been a pitiable object – for she had caught a cold on the journey and had hardly taken possession of her lodgings, before she was again confined to her bed, and suffering under severe and constant pain; and all this amongst strangers with the absolute necessity of having a regular nurse, and finances at that moment particularly unfit to meet any extraordinary expense . . . she had been particularly fortunate in her nurse, as a sister of her landlady, a nurse by profession, and who had always a home in that house when unemployed, chanced to be at liberty just in time to attend her . . . 'Every body's heart is open, you know, when they have recently escaped from severe pain, or are recovering the blessing of health, and nurse Rooke thoroughly understands when to speak. She is a shrewd, intelligent, sensible woman . . . call it gossip if you will; but when nurse Rooke has half an hour's leisure to bestow on me, she is sure to have something to relate that is entertaining and profitable, something that makes one know one's species better . . .' Anne . . . replied 'I can easily believe it. Women of that class have great opportunities and if they are intelligent may be well worth listening to.'

Nurse Rooke may sound indiscreet by modern standards but her behaviour probably reflects the problems of making a living as a freelance nurse. Gossiping with someone like Mrs Smith would be one way of finding out who else was ill and securing recommendations to her friends. But Nurse Rooke's behaviour may also indicate a sensitivity to the importance of nurses' amusing or entertaining their patients, of raising their spirits as well as caring for their physical needs, at a period when carers may have had little else to offer. She is clearly well liked by Mrs Smith.

Nurse Rooke was employed as a live-in servant for particular episodes of illness. When she was not working, she stayed with her sister who kept lodgings for the better-off classes. From the way Anne Elliott and Mrs Smith talk about her, she was obviously thought of as a social inferior, a paid companion rather than an equal. At the same time, she is clearly a superior class of person to Sarah Gamp. This ambiguous status is a marked feature of private duty nurses, who seem to have occupied a marginal role between their employers and the rest of the household staff, rather like that of the governesses. Her work was supported by other servants but, as an employee, she was not the equal of the family members. Donnison (1977: 141) refers to the uncertainty at a later period about whether she should dine with the family or with the servants and Maggs (1986) has noted the questions over her eligibility as a marriage partner for the son of a middle-class household which formed a potent theme in late Victorian popular fiction. Was this a legitimate aspiration or would it merely lead to her seduction and abandonment?

What is perhaps more important is that these structural conditions made the private duty nurse a more specialized care provider than the handywoman. She was also more likely to be working for a client with the resources to purchase medical services so that her work was at least partly defined by whatever passed as orthodox medicine.

These women had their counterparts in the voluntary hospitals. Although there was some internal promotion, sisters and the matron tended to be separately recruited from more elevated social backgrounds than the ordinary nurses. Sisters at St Bartholomew's in the 1830s were described as 'widows in reduced circumstances' and 'persons who have lived in a respectable rank of life'. At St Thomas's in the 1850s they had often been head servants in gentlemen's families. Their status is caught by this later memoir of Guy's Hospital at the same period.

> It appears to have been the custom at all times for each ward to have the benefit of supervision by a separate sister who, in addition to the care of the sick should have the charge of the ward stores and also be the medium of communication between the patients and the medical staff. It . . . was the practice to select for this office respectable females who, previous to their appointment had experience of household work, been upper servants in private families, or been engaged in the capacity of nursing the sick out of doors, and not unfrequently the post was filled by one of the ordinary nurses whose promotion was merited from length of service and presumed suitability. (*Guy's Hospital Reports* (1871): 541–3. Quoted by Williams 1980: 60)

The matron was a senior administrative officer in most hospitals. This advertisement is for a post at Leeds General Infirmary in 1852.

Candidates for this office are required to be free from the care

of a family, of middle age, active, and of good address,
qualified to keep an account of the disbursements and other
matters in the house department; it is necessary that she be
staid, sober, and discreet, mild, and humane disposition, at the
same time possessed of firmness to rule the household; it is also
desirable that she be experienced in the management of a
family and the duties of a sick room. (Woodward 1974: 30)

This is the sort of position that might attract the widow of a
marginal member of the middle classes, such as a clergyman or an
army officer, with the experience of managing a large Victorian
household rather than necessarily of nursing the sick.

In most workhouses, the nurses were supervised by the matron.
She was usually the master's wife and his official deputy.
Workhouse masters were commonly drawn from the ranks of
retired non-commissioned officers in the Army so that one is here
dealing with people of rather more humble origins (Crowther
1981: 116, 125). The matron, as in the voluntary hospitals, was
primarily an administrator. This description of her work is from
the Workhouse Infirmaries Report of 1866.

The matron's duties are varied and multiplied. She
superintends the whole internal working of the establishment,
the cleaning, the linen, the food, the cooking, the distribution
of food, the stores, etc. and in the discharge of these duties has
as much as an active person can properly do. But in many
workhouses she is expected to superintend the nursing and
bedding and other questions relating to the sick. (Quoted by
Abel-Smith 1960: 15–16)

Notice the order of priority.

It would probably be a mistake to draw too strong a distinction
between handywomen and private nurses. Some handywomen
would certainly have had middle-class clients for midwifery
(Donnison 1977: 59) and very possibly for services like the laying-
out of the dead. There was clearly some mobility both socially and
sectorally, between employment and self-employment. A young
woman might plausibly begin as a hospital servant, become a
hospital nurse, leave on marriage, work as a handywoman to
support her family, go into private nursing as a young widow and
finish as a hospital sister. But the social distinctions are important:
private nurses were integrated into the service of the affluent while
handywomen were autonomous workers among the poor. Private
nurses were likely to command other servants while handywomen
laboured on their own or in partnership with other family
members.

Treatment assistants

We have seen that, in the first half of the nineteenth century, the boundary between nursing and domestic service was less clear-cut than it was to become later. But nursing was also to acquire a technical component to its work, as an administrator of medically prescribed treatments. To understand this aspect of the process we need to examine the other side of the occupation's territory, its frontier with medicine. We must in particular consider the work of the apothecary and his assistants and of the apprentice physicians and surgeons.

The apothecaries were often the only salaried medical attendants in a voluntary hospital. Since the early seventeenth century, their guild had successfully enlarged the scope of its work from compounding and supplying medications to advice, prescription and diagnosis. They were an important source of medical care to the middle classes, who were looking for a reasonably reliable practitioner but could not afford the fees of a physician. With the passage of the Apothecaries Act 1815, they became the first of the medical occupations to establish a recognizably modern form of education and registration. Although regarded as social inferiors, they were ultimately to be united with the physicians and surgeons when the medical profession acquired its current shape under the Medical Act 1858, which created the predecessors of the General Medical Council. In the hospitals the apothecary would be responsible for the daily bleedings, scarifyings, cuppings, and blisterings, for the supervision of baths and electrical treatment, and for the maintenance of the surgical instruments, in addition to making up, dispensing and administering the prescribed medications.

During the 1820s, the hospitals also began to be peopled by medical students and junior medical attendants. This resulted from new examination requirements by the College of Surgeons and the Society of Apothecaries. We shall look at the background to these in more detail shortly but part of the consequence was that these new grades of hospital staff came to supplement and eventually take over much of the apothecary's work. At the Royal Devon and Exeter Hospital, for instance, a nurse would help

> with dressings, but only in fetching tins of warm water with which the doctor cleaned the wounds. She was allowed to apply either a bread or linseed poultice but 'as soon as dressings of lotion or lint were ordered, the pupil will take charge' . . . if the state of the patient was such that someone had to sit up all night, it was not the nurse who did so but a pupil. (Hawker 1985: 43–4)

The pupils here were apprenticed to the physicians, surgeons or apothecary. In effect, the forerunners of modern nurses were more like domestic servants because the precursors of modern doctors were performing what would now be regarded as relatively low-level technical procedures and routine treatments, although, at the time, many of them may have been thought to be highly innovative.

How should we assess the quality of nursing care in the early years of the nineteenth century? By modern standards much of it seems basic, primitive and unsophisticated. It may be fairer, however, to judge this care by the standards of its own time. Much of the critical comment on early nineteenth century nursing comes from the writings of reformers like Charles Dickens, Louisa Twining and Florence Nightingale. Some of their descriptions still have an undeniable power to shock and appal. At the same time their judgements would not have been possible without some conception of how nursing care could be given in a more humane fashion. If one relies on hospital records as evidence, then it is important to remember that complaints leave more traces. When a hospital dismissed a nurse for drunkenness, this would generate a series of documents while good work went unreported. It may be just as significant to observe that nurses were dismissed at all, which suggests that hospital administrators were trying to set a positive standard for their staff.

The greatest problem in summarizing early nineteenth century health care is breaking the constraints of present-day assumptions about nursing and medicine. Sick people were nursed by a wide variety of attendants, paid and unpaid, women and men, skilled and unskilled. These attendants provided a range of care which covered basic physical needs, the moral welfare of the patient and some rudimentary treatments. Within this spectrum, the paid nurse, whether at home or in hospital, would mostly have given the elementary physical care that a patient in other circumstances might have received from an amateur family member or personal servant. There was very little technical content. Nurses were drawn from the classes in domestic service and their work was of little interest to anyone other than their immediate employer. While contemporaries were unhappy about the standards of some of the care provided by nurses, especially in the workhouses, it is far from clear that abuse was either systematic or widespread. Nursing care reflected the expectations of the society in which it was given and the limited technology available. The indeterminacy of the occupation's boundaries reflected the limited degree of specialization in the general organization of pre-industrial and early industrial employment.

Chapter two

The Revolution in Nursing

The first evidence of widespread dissatisfaction with the way in which sick people were provided with nursing care dates from the 1830s. It is important to recognize, however, that this evidence does not come from either nurses or patients. Both were likely to belong to classes of the population who leave few written records of their own, even if they were not actually illiterate. The complaints come from two particular sources. One was a group of physicians and surgeons who were introducing new ways of practising medicine that were radically changing the whole nature of hospitals. The other was a circle of well-connected philanthropists whose criticisms expressed both the reforming spirit of evangelical Christianity and a growing concern about the fragility of social order under the stresses of industrialization and urbanization. These two factions had rather different visions for the future of nursing but their combined influence transformed the standards expected from care providers in the home or in institutions.

The rise of the hospital

To understand the changing environment in which nursing care was being given, we need to retrace our steps a little to consider how medical practice had been developing since the end of the eighteenth century among the elite practitioners who were later to join into the modern profession of medicine. Before this time, their work had been only loosely linked to hospitals. These might, as in Edinburgh and Leiden, be places where a medical education happened to be given but they were not centres of research and expertise in the way they are today.

Until the beginning of the nineteenth century, the development of medical knowledge took place in two ways: the elaboration of nosologies, or systems for classifying symptoms, and speculation about the nature of pathology, often attributing all disorders to a single cause treatable by a single remedy or set of remedies. The literate physicians whose writings dominate our image of medicine in this period were encouraged to work in this fashion by the nature of their relationship with their patients. The physicians were the servants of wealthy patrons who had a keen amateur interest in medicine. Since the physicians did not have an effective legal monopoly on the provision of medical treatment, they were forced to compete with each other and with a great variety of irregular healers to attract patients. Each doctor had an incentive to emphasize the novelty of his ideas and their difference from those of his competitors in order to win business. At the same time, the basis of the doctor's appeal would be limited by the opinions of his prospective patients. The emphasis on deriving medical theories from ancient Greek or Roman authors, for example, reflected the prestige attached to that learning by the educated classes among whom the physicians worked.

Since none of these rival systems of medical knowledge had more than a limited technical success, patients' main criterion for judging their treatment was the extent to which they believed that they had received any benefit from their physicians' work. Thus the doctor's manner and his ability to impress patients had a great influence on his prospects of employment. Many of the blood-curdling remedies of this period were accepted by patients because of the way they symbolically dramatized the physician's healing power. Other doctors might place more stress on the niceties of courtly behaviour, cultivating their wit, dress and style in order to encourage patients to identify and value them as gentlemen whose competence and reputation could be assumed from these outward signs (Jewson 1974).

One result of this way of organizing practice was that medicine lagged behind in the dramatic development of the natural sciences during the seventeenth century, despite individual contributions like Harvey's work on the circulation of the blood (Shryock 1979). Writing in the 1620s, Francis Bacon had spelt out the modern vision of science as a collective, co-operative and collegial enterprise where knowledge would advance by the free and open sharing of ideas, discoveries and techniques within a democratic community of scholars. Although there remains much historical debate on the extent to which this was, and, indeed, has ever been, fully realized, it is a vision in sharp contrast to the individualism, jealousy and competitiveness of seventeenth and eighteenth century medicine. Perhaps the most notorious example of this was the secrecy in which the Chamberlen family kept obstetric forceps for some one hundred and twenty-five years in order to preserve an advantage over their competitors (Aveling 1887).

Medical practice of this kind had little use for nurses as such. These elite practitioners might have assistants, servants or apprentices, like the masters of any craft. But healing was a personal art which demanded little in the way of institutional support.

This style of work first began to change in France after the revolution of 1789. Until then, the provision of hospitals had been dominated by the Catholic church. Before effective treatments were available, a good deal of nursing work inevitably involved ministering to the spiritual comfort of patients for whom little else could be done. Consequently both hospital and home nursing were matters of concern to religious interests. At the same time, it meant that they sometimes got caught up in conflicts provoked by the process of secularization that has marked modern societies. In this case, the close association between the hospitals and the church meant that they were initially closed by the Revolutionary Government as part of its attack on organized conservative opposition.

But, just as the English state had found in the sixteenth century, the new French regime was forced to recognize that the suppression of church-based systems of care and welfare left a vacuum which had to be filled by secular equivalents if the government were to command popular support. The revolutionaries reopened the hospitals under state ownership as part of a general plan to expand health and welfare facilities for the poor. This policy continued after the restoration of the monarchy and by 1822 the hospitals of Paris were caring for about 15,000 patients at any one time, some five times as many as were in all the voluntary hospitals of England and Wales (Waddington 1973: 212).

Such comparisons are not entirely straightforward because the Paris hospitals seem to have been admitting some patients who would have figured in Poor Law rather than voluntary hospital statistics. The essential point is that doctors now had access for the first time to very large numbers of poor people who lacked the power or resources to resist their all too often fatal role in the advance of medical knowledge. The mortality rates were easily twice those quoted for English voluntary hospitals. Many of the surgeons, in particular, had developed their skills during the revolutionary wars.[1] Under lay control, experimental medicine could be practised in the French hospitals without the old constraints of Catholic moral teaching.

Such operations were not without their critics, even in Paris, but their tragic results for individual patients paved the way for major advances in therapeutic technique and the understanding of human biology. Of equal importance was the free availability of corpses for dissection. At a time when the English medical colleges only had access to the bodies of a handful of executed criminals each year, their French counterparts in public hospitals had the right to dissect all cases terminating fatally under their care, unless the relatives could pay immediately for a funeral. As a result, diagnoses in life could readily be compared with signs *post mortem*. There were also many more opportunities to observe the process of childbirth. At the Hôpital des Cliniques, the first two students to arrive were allowed to assist the delivery while any others could sit and watch. With an average of two births a day, a good practical knowledge of midwifery could be acquired within a very short period.

In the first decades of the nineteenth century, doctors flocked to Paris in order to learn from this new style of medicine. There were estimated to be 200 English students of anatomy alone in the city in 1828 (Waddington 1973: 224).

Medicine, then, slowly began to become an occupation based upon a scientific model of research rather than on ancient learning and armchair speculation. This new style of practice brought conflicts with traditional institutions. The doctors wanted to use hospitals as locations for studying collections of bodies, living or dead, organized so as to group like cases and differentiate unlike. Admission would be based on the value of a patient's condition for teaching or research purposes rather than on subscribers' patronage. This principle was reflected in the development of a new generation of London hospitals, including University College, Charing Cross and St Mary's, under medical control and directed specifically towards making patients more readily available for teaching or research.

It is important not to think that British medicine changed its way of working suddenly and dramatically. The process of reorganization went on throughout the nineteenth century and only slowly affected lower-status branches of medical work and peripheral regions of the United Kingdom. Tools like stethoscopes, thermometers and pulse watches may not have been routinely used in general practice till the 1850s. Nevertheless, this transformation of medical knowledge in the elite metropolitan institutions had repercussions for the whole division of labour in the care of the sick.

In its initial stages the new style of medicine had placed great emphasis on the direct investigation of the patient by the doctor in order to identify and chart the course of the underlying disease. As the classification of diseases became more clearly defined, however, medical interest shifted towards using this knowledge in a rational search for better treatments. Patient care was now more a matter of identifying the presence of a disease whose course would be predictable, at least in terms of the stages which it went through if not the speed. It was an uneconomic and uninteresting use of the doctor's time simply to observe progress, although it was increasingly important to know when particular things were happening so that appropriate interventions could be made.

There was, then, a gap for a reliable observer who could use the new knowledge to observe disease and to notify the doctor at those points when his contribution would be indicated. This was partly filled by the doctor's assistants or apprentices, whom we met in the previous chapter. Medical education increasingly involved students in spending periods of time on the wards monitoring the condition of patients and administering routine treatments. But this was not a particularly efficient solution to the problem since the students were, by their nature, transients who could not be relied upon to provide continuous and systematic cover. However the doctors' other existing subordinates in the hospital, the nurses, were too poorly educated to discharge the responsibilities of a more sophisticated medical treatment. The doctors faced the same difficulties in the home setting. Even in better-off homes where the care might involve women family members, with some general education, as well as nurse servants, the frontline responsibility rested on well-meaning amateurs.

What seems to have happened is that the doctors began, initially in a rather haphazard and unsystematic way, to improve the education, conditions, and social status of the various grades of nursing staff. At the Royal Cornwall Infirmary in Truro, for example, the house surgeon rather than the matron was appointing nurses by the 1830s and was responsible for granting leave of absence or permission to stay out late (Andrews 1975: 18). In 1835, the Royal Devon and Exeter Hospital had appointed its first 'operation nurse' specifically to care for surgical patients (Hawker 1987: 148). Ward nurses were gradually distinguished from servants. The Nursing Committee of Salisbury Infirmary recommended in 1856, for instance, that 'in future the wards be cleaned and scoured by persons engaged for that purpose and your nurses kept in every particular distinct from the servants of the establishment' (Woodward 1974: 33). Sisters began to be recruited on a supernumerary basis so that they could learn the role before taking over a ward of their own. Their accommodation was upgraded, meals were provided and rates of pay rose. Rosenberg (in press: 213) reports similar developments in the United States from about 1840.

Nursing, then, was already experiencing changes as a result of new medical demands before the Crimean War and the activities of the Nightingale Fund from the 1860s. But it was also being affected by wider social changes in the relationship between the rich and poor in early Victorian Britain.

Nursing as social control

These changes reflected the evolution of new problems of order and forms of social control under the impact of industrialization. The term 'social control' often confuses people who are unfamiliar with sociological ideas. It is not a pathology of particularly oppressive or repressive types of society. Properly understood, it refers to responses to the problem, which all groups face, of maintaining a sufficient degree of order for members to plan and co-ordinate their daily lives so that the group can reproduce itself and survive through time. The precise means which are employed to achieve this goal can, and do, vary greatly, reflecting different types and combinations of incentives and sanctions. We may want to compare and evaluate the choices which are made in particular places at particular times but no society can function without some system of regulation. Even anarchist communes prove to have powerful but unofficial means of controlling their members' behaviour.

One of the most significant contributions of sociology and anthropology to the study of illness and disease has been to see them as forms of social deviance (Parsons 1952: 428–79, Aubert and Messinger 1958, Goffman 1969, Dingwall 1977a). To the extent that sickness is not regarded as an intentional or motivated act, it has different consequences from crime or sin. Nevertheless, it represents a potentially disruptive and destabilizing force in social relationships, since the sick are unable to perform roles on which others may depend. As such it attracts the attention of control agencies. In modern societies, medicine and nursing are among the occupations which help to define what will be socially accepted as normal experiences of the human body and their permissible expressions in behaviour. They also offer the means for returning the deviant to normality or, at least, limiting the impact of their disorder on others.

As we saw at the beginning of Chapter 1, the social control of illness and disease in 1800 was a highly fragmented affair. But it is important to remember that most social activities were similarly decentralized. Both civil and criminal justice relied mainly on local administration within loose national frameworks and there was a great deal of variation from one community to another. Many offences or disputes were dealt with entirely by informal means (Thompson 1968: 66–83, 1971: Stevenson 1977: Quaife 1979: 186–224, cf. Roberts 1979). In the economic sphere, most production was carried out in household groups of fewer than a dozen active members. Larger work groups would be found only in establishments of great families or a few specialized trades like building, mining or shipping. Many workers, especially in rural areas, were relatively unspecialized with income from agricultural production or casual daily labouring being supplemented by earnings from 'putting out' work. This system involved entrepreneurs, particularly in the woollen industry, supplying raw materials and co-ordinating their movements between various households which performed different aspects of the productive process (Laslett 1983: 1–21).

The attempt to describe, explain and evaluate the changes wrought in this way of life by the Industrial Revolution has been a major preoccupation of historians and other social scientists for decades. It would be impossible here to synthesize the relevance of that literature to the analysis of health care in any comprehensive fashion. Nevertheless, certain aspects of this transformation are particularly significant. Two of these are the greatly accelerated movement of population from the countryside to the city and of work from the household to the factory. These had considerable implications for the nature of social control.

Contemporary authors were deeply concerned by what they saw as a collapse of social discipline in the more anonymous environment of towns and cities. Industrialization and urbanization were thought to have destroyed the traditional network of relationships that had maintained harmony and stability. Employers and employed no longer worked beside each other, living in the same districts and sharing many leisure activities. The Anglican church had retreated with the growing prosperity of its clergy after the reform of the tithe system in 1759. There were, then, few natural points of contact which might restrain the undisciplined passions of the poor, passions which found expression in civil disorder, drunkenness, hooliganism and crime.

At the same time, habits of order were increasingly essential to factory production. Expensive machines had to be kept running in order to recover their costs and employers could not reconcile this objective with pre-industrial attitudes to time-keeping and absenteeism (Thompson 1967). Drunkenness and horseplay were particular hazards since workers might not only injure themselves but also harm others and damage equipment or disrupt production (Lambert 1975). Thus the new forms of economic organization also entailed a moral reconstruction of society. Conversely, it was only this moral reconstruction that made the economic change possible.

Again, this was a gradual process, especially in areas where production continued to be based in small workshops, like Birmingham or Sheffield (Reid 1976, Hopkins 1982). In the course of the nineteenth century, however, such concerns led to many experiments in the regulation of working-class life. Traditional sports, fairs and festivals were either abolished or stripped of what middle-class opinion thought of as their wilder elements. Prize-fighting, for instance, gave way to rule-governed boxing. New leisure activities were offered through mechanics' institutes, cheap concerts and temperance clubs, as alternatives to drinking in the ale-house or gin palace (Donajgrodzki 1977). Attempts were made at soaking up disposable income into thrift associations, insurance schemes and provident funds (Supple 1974, Yeo 1979). The overall objective was 'the administration of a cultural lobotomy and the implantation of a new morally superior lobe' (Storch 1977: 139).

The regulation of health was an integral part of these activities. On the one hand, epidemic disease, like the cholera outbreaks of 1832 and 1848, was as much a threat to social order as the riots around the Reform Act of 1832 or the Chartist agitation of the 1840s. On the other, the laws of hygiene were a further means of imposing discipline on an area of working-class life. The control of social behaviour was as important as the control of infections.

This period saw a great proliferation in the techniques of social control. The factory itself offered one model in its idea of collecting people in one, physically-bounded location for a common purpose, and then minutely classifying them according to their role in the division of labour. These principles were reflected in what has been called the 'discovery of the asylum' (Rothman 1971), the erection of prisons, workhouses and other specialized institutions for the socially deviant where they might learn habits of order and discipline. The conceptual changes in medicine which led to the reorganization of existing hospitals and the construction of new ones in the early Victorian period were driven as much by these ideas as by any simple change in medical technology (Foucault 1973).

But asylums are an inefficient means of re-making a society. If they are made too attractive they undermine the incentives to comply with social discipline. If they are too repressive, those marked for incarceration may evade it and pose an even greater threat from their rootless nonconformity. The same considerations apply equally to the itinerant beggar and the carrier of smallpox. Consequently, those concerned for social order were drawn inexorably into the search for ways of regulating ordinary activities and relationships that would be more subtle, more sensitive and more precisely calculated than the crude isolation of the proven deviant (Donzelot 1980, Foucault 1979).

Organized philanthropy played an important part in this movement. As Donzelot (1980: 55–8) points out, it can be a way to control sections of the population without the open and coercive use of the state's power. It has two principal modes of action: *assistance*, which is the private provision of economic aid to the needy so that eligibility is a matter of discretion rather than of right, and moral conditions can be applied apparently as a matter of the philanthropist's choice rather than the state's definition; and *medical-hygienism*, direct involvement with the people who had shown themselves physically or morally ill-equipped to maintain a respectable life. Those who had failed to meet the standards of private behaviour set out by the philanthropists would be denied assistance and abandoned to the meagre provision of the state. Both here and outside they would remain a target for medical-hygienic action, in the visiting of prisons, workhouses, hospitals or homes.

Thus, a particularly important element in the process of moral reconstruction was direct contact between members of different classes so that the poor could model their behaviour at first hand on the living example of their betters. It was an attempt to generalize the workplace discipline imposed on domestic servants in the middle-class home.

> The female servants in your household, whom you have taken and instructed in their respective duties – whose manners you have softened – who have learnt from you how to manage a household – who have caught up from you, insensibly, lessons of vast utility . . . if then it were possible . . . for the ladies of England to extend that influence over all classes of the poor . . . I really believe the blessing to this nation would be inestimable.
> (Rev. J.S. Brewer, 1855, *Lectures to Ladies on Practical Subjects*. Quoted by Summers, 1979: 40–1)

This theory led to the development of a number of schemes which organized middle- and upper-class women to visit the homes of the poor as missionaries for ideals of Christian self-discipline, sobriety and domestic economy. It is important not to trivialize these as the leisure activities of idle spinsters. While these may have been the people with time available, the work was undertaken out of a positive sense of duty as a deliberate alternative to playing music, eating chocolates or reading frivolous novels. As Summers (1979: 39–40) notes, some of it also had a utilitarian element in recruiting potential domestic servants.

Some of these visiting schemes included the provision of home nursing. The best-known of these are the Protestant Sisters of Charity (founded in 1840), the Sisterhood of the Holy Cross (1845), and the Sisterhood of Mercy of Devonport and Plymouth (1848), which were amalgamated in 1856, and the St John's House Training Institution for Nurses (1848). The first of these was founded by Elizabeth Fry, who came from a prominent Quaker family. This sect had developed a strong tradition of social activism since the accusations of an unpatriotic refusal to contribute to the nation provoked by its members' pacifism during the Napoleonic Wars (Fears 1977, 1978). Miss Fry had been to visit the hospital at Kaiserwerth in Germany run by Pastor Fliedner, whom she had known since the 1820s, and his deaconesses, eleven years before a similar trip by Florence Nightingale. She was equally inspired by this example of a Christian community which also provided home nursing in the locality. On returning to London, she prompted her sisters and daughters to establish a similar association. The other groups all had High Anglican connections and owed more to Catholic models: indeed a number of their members eventually converted to the Roman church. These strong religious identifications caused a certain amount of rivalry and also generated hostility to their work in secular institutions. St John's House, for instance, took over the nursing service at King's College Hospital, with which it had been closely linked, in 1856 but the connection was severed in 1867 over the decision of Mary Jones, the superintendent, and her nurses to take open religious vows and set up their own altar with an exposed sacrament.

A closer look at the St John's Institution allows us to examine exactly what was meant by 'nursing' in this context. There were three grades of membership: probationers and nurses, who were trained for both private and hospital work but were also expected to assist with domestic duties, receiving board, lodging and wages; sisters, who trained the probationers and visited the sick and aged poor, receiving no wages and paying for their own living expenses; and associate sisters, who did not live in the house but gave general support to its work. Candidates for training were supposed to be churchgoers but they seem to have been drawn largely from the servant classes. The quality of their education should not be overstressed. It was essentially practical in nature and provided by the sisters, who had, themselves, no specific training beyond the, not inconsiderable, skills in domestic management appropriate to their upper middle-class backgrounds. The sisters set the spiritual tone:

> It was not just a question of replacing drunken Sarah Gamps with a more respectable class of women who could be trusted to cook, clean and attend to the patients' physical requirements. No matter how satisfactorily these tasks were carried out, the patients were not being properly cared for if their souls were not receiving the same degree of attention. (Summers 1983: 35)

Orders like St John's House, then, actually seem to have been recruiting from the handywoman class in the same way as the voluntary hospitals were.

It would be a mistake to claim too much in the way of practical effect for the sisterhoods. As Baly (1987: 4) points out, the nurses earned their keep by being sent out to private employment. The care of the sick poor was something which they did between paying engagements. The precarious economies of financing home nursing on a charitable basis also forced the same compromise on later, more secular schemes, generally to the detriment of their service to the poor (Baly 1987: 20).

But the model of the sisterhoods did make an important contribution to the reconceptualization of nursing. In contrast to the ordinary duties of the hospital nurse or the independent handywoman, the work of the sisterhood nurse took on an explicitly moral character. The secular spirit of medical modernization was complemented by the spiritual concerns of the order. Dying patients could be helped to salvation and living patients brought to reflect on their past behaviour, recognizing the generosity of a society which offered them this assistance and opportunity for a new start. The sisterhoods began to break the cultural link between the handywoman and her patients. Although the nurses still performed a rather undifferentiated set of tasks, they clearly had a much more regular occupation. Moreover, they were not, as the handywomen were, merely occupants of a traditional role who were mobilized by the sick person and his or her immediate caretakers. Sisterhood nursing was organized by and accountable to social superiors. Thus the type of deviance represented by sickness was ceasing to be a purely local concern but being brought within a wider framework of social control. The nurses, disciplined like domestic servants, bore the same discipline into the homes or wards where they worked.

Similar medical-hygienic concerns are also evident in the pressures for change that were brought to bear on the workhouses where the sick and poor received most of their care. These institutions were, however, much less responsive to change.

The workhouses had been less affected by the developments in medical practice. The Poor Law reforms of 1834 reflected the belief of Edwin Chadwick, one of their principal sponsors, that sanitary engineering was the real answer to disease. Consequently, the main emphasis of the legislation was on restricting medical profiteering and deterring extravagant treatment. Appointments were not restricted to holders of recognized qualifications and were made by a process of competitive tendering for small annual contracts. In some areas, the medical officer had to purchase all his drugs and appliances out of the fixed sum. Poor Law appointments were usually held on a part-time basis by practitioners with insufficient private patients to sustain them or as a means of preventing potential competitors from getting a toe-hold in the locality (Loudon 1987: 245–6).

Poor Law medical practice was closely associated with the discipline of the workhouse. It was the medical officer who determined which inmates were 'able-bodied' and required a corrective regime designed to deter them from idleness. The medical officer also had to decide whether inmates who broke workhouse rules were fit enough to withstand the resulting punishments. All of this generated a good deal of paperwork which, together with the constant accounting to the board of guardians, made the practice unattractive to the medical profession. Some medical officers were conscientious and caring, others were indifferent, often hiring assistants to carry out this work, while yet others were cruel and corrupt. Those who were critical found their contracts were not renewed. Again, however, there is evidence of gradual improvement. Tendering was abolished in 1842, although medical officers remained on annual contracts till 1854. More importantly, in 1842 the Poor Law commissioners stipulated that medical officers must be qualified in both medicine and surgery and from 1858 local guardians could engage only practitioners licensed under the Medical Act of that year. As procedures of some clear value became available – smallpox vaccinations, midwifery and some surgery – guardians were allowed to offer fees to encourage their medical officers to provide those services. There is at least an argument that the results of these policies did protect the poor from over-treatment with ineffective or harmful medications and from enthusiastic surgery and, by making improved diet the most readily available prescription, inadvertently meant that malnourished patients received the most useful assistance then available (Crowther 1981: 160).

On the other hand, they also meant that medical advances were slow to percolate into the workhouse sick wards and that the medical officers do not generally seem to have become involved in the pressure for change until the late 1860s. Most of the nursing, then, continued to be performed by other inmates. It was their conduct that aroused the concern of reformers. Again, however, this seems to have focused less on the limitations of the physical care than on the way in which it subverted the reformers' ideal of the workhouse as a site for moral regeneration.

Workhouse visiting initially encountered much greater opposition than home visiting. Summers (1979: 48) points out that one of the less recognized effects of the 1834 Poor Law reform had been to break the traditional relationships of patronage and dependency between women from wealthy families and their poor clients. The new Poor Law was administered by the small tradesmen and retailers who had been left behind in the cities by the migration of better-off households to the suburbs. Whereas the governors of voluntary hospitals and the trustees of home visiting schemes were men who shared the background values of the women philanthropists, and were thus vulnerable to their social leverage, guardians tended to come from a lower class and were concerned both with the burden of property taxation and with the need to draw a firm line beneath their own fragile respectability by stigmatizing paupers (Abel-Smith 1964). Louisa Twining[2] wrote an article in 1857 complaining:

> Everywhere we hear of gentlemen resigning their posts as Guardians because of the opposition of the majority, whose ignorance and vulgarity cannot be tolerated by them. It is the same in the country as in the towns; the ill-educated and narrow-minded have the upper hand. (Quoted by Summers 1979: 48)

Although this reflects the characteristic ungenerosity of the committed reformer, it conveys the obstacles to any improvement in the general treatment of paupers. The Poor Law commissioner and the local guardians emphasized the reform of inmates by the negative techniques of deterrence: their opponents thought that paupers should also be given positive incentives to change their way of life.

The sick were no exception. It was hard to shift Parliament from its view that the only people in the workhouses were the indolent unemployed, although by 1861 they were caring for something like 50,000 sick people as compared with 11,000 in the voluntary hospitals (Abel-Smith, 1964: 46). As we noted in the previous chapter, most of their care was provided by other inmates. Although a few of the larger urban workhouses had begun appointing paid nurses to assist the matrons in supervising the paupers caring for the sick from the mid-1840s onwards, by 1866 the 40 workhouses in London employed only 142 nurses to attend approximately 21,250 sick and infirm patients. Two workhouses accounted for 35 of the nurses, leaving 107 to care for 18,000 patients in the others (Abel-Smith 1964: 55).

Both reformers and later official investigations have left ample evidence of the limitations of this practice, although such writers would, of course, often have been motivated to emphasize the deficiencies. As the Manchester guardians observed, the care that was offered was probably as much as the working poor could afford for themselves from the handywoman type of provider. The result was a mixture of kindness, squalor, superstition, corruption and abuse (Crowther 1981: 166–7).

Matched against the standards of the lady reformers, however, the system amounted to an acquiescence in poverty and disease. The poor were punished but offered no hope of redemption, in this world or the next. Their visitors brought small material comforts which, if nothing else, might become currency to bribe officers or other inmates for better treatment, and a message of support. If the visitors' pressures were relatively ineffective before the late 1860s, it was because local guardians were suspicious that the result of yielding would compromise the principle of less eligibility and the national Poor Law board had not yet felt the full weight of their lobbying.

Looking at the thirty years or so before the establishment of the Nightingale School at St Thomas's Hospital in 1860, we can, then, already discern significant changes in the social environment for nursing care. On the one hand, developments in medical practice were leading doctors to demand different qualities and knowledge from those who actually spent long periods of time at the bedside. The patient population of the voluntary hospitals was changing as doctors sought to treat or study patients with acute conditions. Alongside this was the growing interest of a rather heterogeneous body of women reformers who were 'less concerned to ask whether a disease had been cured or an epidemic checked, than to ask whether a stay in hospital would degrade an individual, or make her or him a better human being' (Summers 1983: 50).

One problem for the medical-hygienic reformers, however, was the limited availability of suitable personnel. An important element in generating support for change was the way in which the standard of respectability crossed social classes, as studies of the RSPCA (Harrison 1967) and NSPCC (Behlmer 1982) have shown. The middle and upper classes were challenged to live up to the genteel values they prescribed for the working class. Thus a middle-class woman's duty was primarily to her own family and only secondarily to social service. One of the grounds on which the nursing sisterhoods were frequently attacked was their subversion of family loyalties. Even unmarried women had an obligation to parents or siblings in times of need. Part of the conflict between Florence Nightingale and her family seems to have revolved around her reluctance to share in caring for her sister during a period of poor health in the 1840s. The demographic surplus of women in the nineteenth century was much less readily mobilized than many writers have supposed. Philanthropic activity could not be sustained on the voluntary efforts of well-born ladies alone.

The physicians and the philanthropists converged on the same set of potential candidates to implement their programmes, in the hospital and in the home. These were the 'respectable' strata of working-class women from whom the better sort of domestic servants were recruited. They were people who, it was thought, could be trusted to implement without challenge the directions either of their secular male superiors, the physicians and surgeons, or of their spiritual female superiors, the professional and upper-class women who governed the voluntary associations for whom they worked.

The co-option of working-class women to the task of maintaining order in society is an important theme in Donzelot's (1980) work. In contrast to those feminist historians who have emphasized the attempts to control women, he argues that the nineteenth and early twentieth centuries saw the development of an alliance between women and the state, mediated by the activities of the philanthropists. This remedied some of the material grievances of working-class women in exchange for them accepting a role as bearers and transmitters of social discipline. The ideologies of domesticity and motherhood were intended to act through women to influence the conduct of men. The price on the benefits of family life, in support and personal service to men, was their commitment to the economic and social behaviour necessary to sustain it. Poor women were, for example, denied divorce but offered the legal framework of separation on the theory that a man who was compelled to provide economic support to a family, whether he lived with them or not, would so restrain his behaviour as to maintain secure employment and his acceptability as a companion (cf. McGregor *et al*. 1970: 1–29). The rough edges of working-class life would be smoothed to a pattern of compliance with an upper- or middle-class vision of harmonious social relations. Nursing reform offered not only practical help to women carers but also a stable and respectable alternative to domestic employment.

The price, if it may be so phrased, was the erosion of the independent role of the handywoman. Pre-industrial networks of community organization would give way before the newly constituted occupation with its more explicit and externally imposed discipline. The revolution in nursing was not a revolution of nurses or patients. It was rather a 'revolution of expectations'. The complaints about the quality of care do not seem to bear on any documentable deterioration but more closely reflect the new standards which were being set. Old ways were no longer acceptable to their sponsors and patrons.

Chapter three

The New Model Nurse

One of the great problems for anybody studying the history of nursing in the nineteenth century is to find a way of coming to terms with the powerful and enigmatic figure of Florence Nightingale, a woman who became the stuff of which myths are made even in her own lifetime. In this chapter, however, we shall try to place her in a social context as a woman of her class and time. As we have seen, the care of the sick was already changing in many ways which were ultimately to produce the modern occupation of nursing. Florence Nightingale's work was part of that process and undeniably made a major contribution to its outcome. But that result was a compromise between Miss Nightingale's vision and the realities of mid-Victorian life, values and institutions; a compromise shaped by the hands of many other women and men. The 'New Nurse' turned out to retain a surprisingly large number of features of the old.

Florence Nightingale: woman and myth

The difficulty of assessing the contribution of Florence Nightingale to nursing reform in the nineteenth century is that so much of the writing about her has been biographical rather than historical. This has, perhaps, been encouraged by the mass of her own papers which present vivid, if often selective, melodramatic and egotistic accounts and judgements of other people and events. Florence Nightingale's life has taken on the function of a 'heroine legend' in nursing, a morality tale to inspire her successors (Whittaker and Oleson 1964). To see her, rather, as part of a social movement is not to detract from her contribution but is to acknowledge the complex relationship between individuals and their circumstances in the making of history.

Thus, some of the more breathless accounts of her early life try to trace Florence Nightingale's mission to nursing in events of her childhood and youth, an attempt in which they are encouraged by her own reconstructions in late middle age. Cook (1913: 14), her first scholarly biographer, puts these in perspective:

> Florence Nightingale is not the only little girl who has been fond of nursing sick dolls or mending them when broken. Other children have tended wounded animals and had their pill-boxes and simples. Much too has been written about Florence's kindness as a child to her poorer neighbours. . . . But thousands of other squires' daughters, before and after her, have done the like.

But she was more than a simple squire's daughter. Her parents are not easily seen as the weak or obstructive figures of their daughter's waspish private portraits. William Nightingale was a rich and well-educated gentleman with a serious interest in travel, scholarship and liberal politics. Although disappointed in his own parliamentary ambitions, he had an important network of friends throughout the reformist intelligentsia of Britain and Europe. Fanny Nightingale was the respected hostess to a salon of politicians and socially concerned intellectuals. The values of this circle were reflected in the 'advanced' quality of education given to the Nightingale daughters. Some of Florence's cruellest comments were reserved for her older sister, Parthenope, whom she caricatured in her letters and diaries as vain and trivial. Parthenope may have taken more pleasure in London society but she was also the author of five novels, essays on agricultural reform and a history of her husband's family. Despite their occasional differences, the sisters appear to have remained on familiar terms until Parthenope's death.

Although it cannot have been easy to sustain good relationships with the sensitive and autocratic Florence, her family actually seem to have been a considerable source of support in her various adventures (Smith 1982: 18–21). If they occasionally opposed her, it may have been less a matter of simple prejudice than of their recognition of her impulsive character and a rationalist suspicion of her mystic religious tendencies.

These religious enthusiasms are an important element in understanding Florence Nightingale's work. They combined the fervour of the time with her intense egotism. She had a strong sense of personal vocation, based on direct conversations with God, that transcended the sectarianism of the sisterhoods. Thus, while her work was permeated with many of the values that we identified in early Victorian philanthropy, their realization was driven by her feeling of speaking and writing with a unique divine authority. Organized religion and Biblical teaching played a subordinate part in this enterprise. Reflecting her Unitarian upbringing, however, her beliefs placed an authentically Protestant emphasis on the importance of performing Christian deeds.

The behaviour which resulted has generated modern assessments of her character which are sharply at odds with the traditional selfless image. Smith, for example, describes her as narcissistic.

> In public she was gracious and ingratiating, immensely productive and politically effective. In private she indulged in bouts of self-depreciation, scorn of others, and guilt of her passion for fame and her destructive use of her allies . . . from childhood Florence was alternately unpredictably wilful and petulant, and a docile seeker of adult approval. (Smith 1982: 22)

This may reflect the difficulty twentieth century scholars sometimes have in taking Victorian religious beliefs seriously. In the terms of our own day, it may be better to see her thinking as an attempt to resolve the guilt of a rich liberal intellectual woman who both enjoyed the privileges of her birth and was tormented by the knowledge of the material and spiritual poverty of those whose labour made her position possible. But, as with other philanthropists, she thought the answer lay in personal work rather than in large-scale social reform. Her judgement in 1873 on another philanthropic activist, Octavia Hill,[1] is revealing.

> Were there one such woman with power to direct the flow of volunteer help nearly everywhere running to waste, in every street of London's East End, almost might the East End be persuaded to become Christian. (Quoted by Cook 1913: 97)

Her interest in service to the community appears to have begun to focus on public health questions during the 1840s. But, again, it is important not to see this as somehow exceptional or unique. Sanitary reform was one of the great political issues of the day and her father's friends were among its leading advocates. A woman with a growing reputation for culture and intelligence could not fail to study the topic if she were to hold her own in conversation. Moreover, it is important to recognize that nursing was only ever one part of Florence Nightingale's interests in health policy. Although she clung ferociously to miasmatic theory, the idea that disease was transmitted by foul air, long past its discrediting in the medical world, she constantly emphasized the prior contribution of environmental measures to promote good health. In her own assessment, sanitary engineering, hospital architecture and health education were all of greater importance than the direct care of the sick. Throughout her life she was a sanitary reformer first and a nursing reformer second.

Nevertheless, there is some evidence of Florence Nightingale's developing concern about nursing during the 1840s. The wife of an American physician who visited the Nightingales in 1844 recorded Florence as expressing a desire to perform 'works of charity in hospitals and elsewhere as Catholic sisters do' (Woodham-Smith 1950: 39). This was followed in 1845 by a plan

> to go to be a nurse at Salisbury Hospital for these few months to learn the 'prax' and then come home and make such wondrous intimacies at West Wellow, under the shelter of a rhubarb powder and a dressed leg . . . . I thought something like a Protestant Sisterhood, without vows, for women of educated feelings might be established. (Letter to Hilary Bonham-Carter quoted by Cook 1913: 44)

The proposal came to nothing against the opposition of her mother and Mrs Fowler, wife of the physician to the Salisbury Infirmary, who were concerned by the moral hazards of the enterprise. We shall analyse such anxieties in more detail later.

But neither of these ideas was wholly revolutionary. As we saw in the previous chapter, the concept of the sisterhood was already established as a socially acceptable form of public service for women from good families. Florence Nightingale's mistake, as far as her family were concerned, may have been to propose going on her own rather than as part of an organized group. The frequent references from around this date to her inspecting hospitals in Britain, Europe, and the Near East do not support the view that her family opposed her intellectual interest in institutional reform. The proposal to spend time at Salisbury Infirmary is linked to her work with local villagers. It may well simply reflect the expectation that educated people living in the country might provide medical advice or treatment to the local poor. Instead of relying on home remedy books, Florence Nightingale seems to have thought she could learn from hospital practice. Her reference to 'rhubarb powder and a dressed leg' recalls Hawker's (1987) description of the work assigned to the physician's apprentice in the 1830s. Nurses may have taken this over by 1845 but the overall impression is more one of an aspiration to perform a traditional duty more effectively than to be an innovator.

Her involvement with the sisterhoods developed over the next few years. She formed an intense friendship with Mary Stanley during a visit to Rome in the winter of 1847 (Woodham-Smith 1950: 56). The two women fell out badly in the Crimea and this may have led to an underestimation of the importance of this connection. Mary Stanley was the daughter of the Bishop of Norwich and sister of a future Dean of Westminster. She was travelling with Henry, later Cardinal, Manning as part of the process of religious exploration that would lead them both into the Catholic church. At the time, however, they were involved with the High Anglican circles which were establishing nursing orders. The two women remained in close contact during the early 1850s. Mary Stanley helped recruit the first party of nurses to go out to the Crimea, including a contingent of nuns provided by Manning. Moreover, he arranged for Florence Nightingale to study with a Catholic nursing order in Paris during 1853, although this was disrupted by her grandmother's death and by an attack of measles. Florence Nightingale also took an independent interest in the Protestant nursing order at Kaiserswerth which had influenced Elizabeth Fry and her associates. She visited the community in 1850 and again in 1851, when she stayed for three months.

These experiences generated a mixed response. On the one hand, she admired the moral force of the sisterhoods. The deaconesses at Kaiserswerth, in particular, were peasant women whose faith disciplined their lives in ways which neutralized the moral suspicion with which the nineteenth century poor were regarded by their social superiors. On the other, Florence Nightingale was unimpressed by the priority given to Godliness over cleanliness, although she never publicly criticized the poor diet and hygiene recorded in her private notes. Simply caring was insufficient unless it was allied to concern for the sanitary conditions of the patient.

The first opportunity to put her theories into practice came when she was appointed Superintendent of an 'Establishment for Gentlewomen during Illness' in August 1853. It was a type of institution that was developing in London at this period to provide accommodation for single middle-class people who needed medical care and had no family at hand, or for patients from out of London. The voluntary hospitals were still mainly for the working class. Of the 10,414 patients recorded by the 1861 census only 157 were grouped as 'professional people' and 14 as 'persons of Rank or Property' (Abel-Smith 1964: 41). The remainder were wage-earners in industry, domestic service or agriculture. If the wealthy wanted treatment by a London consultant they either paid him to travel to them or took a house in London. The less affluent provincial sick, however, took lodgings in the neighbourhood of the great men's consulting rooms, where they could be visited and treated. Private hospital care was not established on any scale until the end of the century.

The patients in Florence Nightingale's care are described as 'governesses and other gentlewomen of narrow means'. Governesses occupied an ambiguous position in Victorian society. Typically, they came from impoverished middle-class backgrounds. Their social status was compromised by the need to earn their own living but their birth made it inappropriate to treat them as servants.[2] This institution offered subsidized accommodation, giving them private care at a price they could afford. Florence Nightingale avoided the stigma of being paid by receiving an allowance from her father and established a regime modelled on the management of sickness in a large household. She was not a deliverer of care but an organizer of others' labour. Her improvements had as much to do with increasing the productivity of the staff and enhancing the sanitary conditions as with directly improving the comfort of the patients. Indeed, she was profoundly suspicious of them and imposed a much stricter discipline on their lives, reducing their diets and rigidly enforcing rules about the length of stay permitted.

As Smith (1982: 13–16) points out, the result was to precipitate an acute state of chaos and a financial crisis. The patients and servants voted with their feet. Within twelve months she seems to have run through two complete sets of servants and there was only one nurse left in employment by August 1854. The bed occupancy never seems to have exceeded 30 per cent. Nevertheless, the council of well-known philanthropists were strongly impressed by her ideas on economy and moral order. There were discussions about her taking over the post of superintendent at King's College Hospital. Cook's (1913: 140–1) account, however, underlines the continuing influence of the sisterhood model. The King's post would allow her to train volunteers, who would necessarily come from affluent backgrounds, over a paid staff of 'farmers' daughters'.

Much as she might personally have resisted the conclusion, it is hard to see Florence Nightingale's contribution to nursing before 1854 as constituting a radical break from the philanthropic approach. Her differences with the sisterhoods are as much a reflection of her sense of having a unique vocation and her Unitarian education as of substance. The language in which she expressed her ideas is less marked by sectarian religiosity and owes a greater debt to secular, scientific work on public health. But she saw the laws of health as part of the Divine ordering of society which it was her duty to interpret and sustain. Thus her vision of who nurses should be and what they should do contained the same elements of discipline as those adopted by the sisterhoods. What was new was the emphasis on the hygienic aspects of their practice. Even these, however, were as much a means to the moral improvement of patients and nurses as an end in themselves, as the Crimean experience shows.

Army nursing: the civilizing mission

As Summers points out (1988: 23–4, 26–7) nobody had considered army nursing as a prime site for the efforts of reformers before 1854. Indeed, the army offered its men and their families a more comprehensive system of medical care than would have been available to any civilian, and its sanitary discipline had protected them during the cholera epidemics of the 1830s and 1840s. Each regiment had its own medical officer and hospital where sick soldiers were nursed by male orderlies detached from the same regiment. These men were not trained as nurses but acquired considerable experience during their service. Soldiers' wives had been employed as nurses since the end of the eighteenth century, and possibly earlier. After 1838, they were not supposed to attend male patients, but they seem to have continued to staff the beds for regimental wives and children that were also provided in the military hospitals. These women, in practice, also seem to have nursed men: at least three applicants for war nursing posts in 1854 claimed to have such experience.

A detailed discussion of the problems of providing medical services in the Crimea can be found in Summers (1988: 30–5). Briefly, most were attributable to the difficulty of mobilizing a peacetime army for its first major European war in half a century. This exposed weaknesses in the co-ordination of medical, supply, and combat arms. Nobody had any realistic idea how many casualties to expect or how long a campaign to plan for. The whole situation was compounded by epidemics of cholera. Snow's research pointing to the water-borne transmission of the disease was only just available and was not fully accepted by the army until 1896. On the nursing side experienced able-bodied orderlies were recalled for combat duties and replaced by inexperienced men who were unfit for active service. They were asked to work in hospitals and casualty stations overflowing with severely injured and sick men and organized on a model designed for small peacetime establishments catering for minor injuries and illnesses. A great deal of the orderlies' time was spent away from their patients, queueing for food, queueing for it to be cooked, queueing for medical supplies and so on. These were failures of command not of the medical department in itself.

Nevertheless, it was the Army Medical Department which became the object of public censure in the reports of W. H. Russell, the war correspondent of *The Times*. These provoked at least two offers of parties of nurses to go out to the Crimea: one from the Rev. Mr Hume, formerly chaplain at Birmingham General Hospital and a man with previous army experience; and one from Lady Maria Forester, who was associated with the Protestant Institution of Nursing Sisters. Both of these were made to War Office officials. Florence Nightingale appears to have become aware of the Forester initiative and taken it over by going directly to politicians with whom she was acquainted and through them to the head of the Army Medical Department. More importantly, she also mobilized an old friendship with Elizabeth Herbert, wife of the Secretary at War, Sidney Herbert, and a member of the Ladies' Committee at the 'Establishment for Gentlewomen'. Through Mrs Herbert, she set up what most biographers have depicted as one of the great coincidences of history, an exchange of letters with the Herberts establishing her leadership of a party of nurses to go out to the Crimea. Smith (1982: 26) shows, from Parthenope Nightingale's correspondence, that an arrangement was reached between Florence and Mrs Herbert, who then dealt with her husband, leading to a carefully orchestrated and apparently spontaneous crossing of Florence's offer to serve and Sidney Herbert's offer of appointment.

The effect was to concentrate power in the hands of the comparatively inexperienced Florence Nightingale, since she refused to accept any leader from the institutions she approached to supply nurses. For the first party, 38 women were engaged: 8 sisters from two High Anglican orders, 6 nurses from St John's House, 5 nuns from each of two Catholic convents and 14 hospital nurses (Summers 1988: 38). The last were selected by Mary Stanley, Elizabeth Herbert and another old friend, Selina Bracebridge. The expedition was initially boycotted by the non-denominational Protestant nursing institution founded by Elizabeth Fry which, Summers (1986: 36) suggests, may have felt snubbed by the usurpation of Maria Forester's initiative.

Looking at the constitution of the party, it is clear that in no sense was it a radical break with the past. The ladies were associated with institutions already taking a leading role in nursing reform while the paid women had considerable experience in the voluntary hospitals. The same pattern is reflected in the composition of a second party which went out about two months later under the leadership of Mary Stanley. The 46 women in this contingent included 21 working women with experience of caring for the sick, 10 ladies and 15 Irish Catholic nuns.

The conflict and intrigue that went on between these groups is an unedifying story which need not concern us here, except perhaps to note the need for a more even-handed treatment of Mary Stanley's group than Florence Nightingale's biographers have usually allowed (Summers 1988: 43–4, 72–4). They were far from being the 'spiritual flirts' of her portrait but included a number of women who were subsequently to make significant contributions. The most notable was probably Jane Shaw Stewart who came from a wealthy Scottish family and had experience of both English and German hospitals before the war. She was later to become superintendent of female nurses at Woolwich military hospital in the early 1860s. But the principal fault of the second party was that they were not under Florence Nightingale's control and there was no great enthusiasm in the Crimea for extending her warrant over them. Our picture has been filtered through her anger and conspiracy to increase her authority. Smith (1982) and Summers (1988: 44–7) provide more detailed accounts of these events.

Of more interest here is the struggle to define what the work of a nurse was and who should do it, a conflict of principles which exacerbated the clashes between the forceful women and men involved. As Summers (1983: 41–2, 47) notes, the Crimea was the arena for an important confrontation between two very different models of the proper relationship between working-class women and their employers. The paid nurses were used to working under ordinary conditions of employment in the open market for labour. Like the women who were employed in mines or factories, they defined their job in fairly practical terms, in this case the physical care of sick or wounded men from their own class. Their relationship with their employers was strictly commercial. The lady members of both parties, however, were used to relating to working-class women as domestic servants, socially and economically dependent upon their mistresses' patronage and, hence, pliable to their standards of conduct. The ladies' view of the civilizing mission of nursing carried little weight with the women engaged for this trip. Their less genteel behaviour was rapidly equated with moral looseness. If the ladies were not to find themselves stigmatized by their own class, out of the same concerns that had obstructed Florence Nightingale's proposed work at Salisbury, they had to establish their dominance and impose their own ideals on their associates.

Their methods were essentially those of the sisterhoods, a re-creation of the discipline of the Victorian household, as Summers shows (1983: 41–2, 44–7). The paid nurses were pressed to act as domestic servants to the ladies as well as caring for the sick. The ladies abandoned their uniforms while insisting the women wore theirs. Paid nurses and ladies ate separately. The women were not permitted access to patients or indeed any significant mobility except under a lady's supervision. Indeed, Summers argues that these were not just the conditions of a resident domestic servant but verged on the system, known to Mary Stanley, devised by a sisterhood running a house for reformed prostitutes.

The result of this treatment was a stream of dismissals on the flimsiest of grounds. Florence Nightingale had sent home thirteen of her original party by Christmas 1854 (Smith 1982:40). Half the paid nurses in Mary Stanley's party lost their posts within eight months and Lady Canning, a selector, wrote from England in the Spring of 1855, 'From experience we learn to mistrust regular hospital nurses and very few of them should be engaged. There is no doubt but that household servants and private nurses after a little teaching answer best' (Summers 1983: 47–8). This policy was enshrined in official regulations by December 1855. Domestic work was prescribed for the paid nurses and they were cautioned:

> It having been found that some of the nurses have believed they
> were to be on an equality with the ladies or sisters, it is
> necessary that they should understand that they will remain in
> exactly the same relative position as that in which they were in
> England. (Quoted in Summers 1983: 48)

Having civilized the nurses, the ladies' next task was to civilize the hospitals.

The picture of filth and squalor drawn by the journalist Russell and by Florence Nightingale is almost certainly exaggerated. Private letters from medical officers to their families emphasize the cleanliness and suitability of the accommodation and the availability of supplies to anyone who understood how to obtain them (Cope 1958: 47). The different judgements may reflect the different standards of the genteel reformers and the professional surgeons. Were hospitals to be compared with the homes of the servant-keeping classes or with army barracks and field service conditions? Was the alleged problem of supply actually the result of an influx of inexperienced medical staff and orderlies who did not know how to work the system? The doctors certainly thought that the cholera epidemics were the result of misfortune rather than mismanagement and there is evidence that they were applying to the best of their ability the theories of the time about the prevention of transmission.

Nevertheless, there is an old sociological dictum that if men define a situation as real, it is real in its consequences. In this case, it was the ladies' definition which was consequential. As Summers (1988: 47–9) shows, they saw a need to improve the cleanliness and supply organization of the hospitals, problems of supervision and co-ordination familiar to them as household managers. In fact, the greater part of the actual work continued to be done by male orderlies and soldiers' wives. The main contribution of the Nightingale party seems to have been to bully, persuade and cajole these auxiliary helpers into performing their tasks more efficiently and to ensure that improved means were available to them in this work through the party's access to private funds for the purchase of extra supplies and equipment. Florence Nightingale, herself, was concerned to limit the presence of women in the hospital in case the men were overindulged and the regime were made so comfortable as to encourage them to stay. She thought that a ratio of two to three female nurses per hundred severely wounded men was about right and that their personal efforts should be concentrated on the dying.

It was only where Miss Nightingale's writ ran less strongly that nurses took on more substantial responsibilities for the administration of medicines and the watching of patients at night (Summers 1988: 49–52). But Victorian notions of proper sexual conduct prevented much involvement in direct care. The female nurses could fan patients, place ice in their mouths or help them turn in bed but they could not, for instance, wash more than a small part of the body surface. Despite the civilian experience of some of the paid nurses with surgical patients, they do not seem to have been permitted to make any contribution to the dressing of wounds. One assistant surgeon's verdict to his parents is particularly telling:

> I did not see Miss Nightingale herself, but I met several others of the 'sympathizers' as we call them . . . . The M.O.s say they are very kind and do a great deal of good but are very much in the way. (Letter of Arthur Henry Taylor, quoted by Cope 1958: 47)

The term 'sympathizers' may give away a great deal. The material improvements to which the Crimean nurses contributed were born out of moral concerns. It was the precise shape of these, however, which underlay many of the conflicts between the nurses' leaders. Florence Nightingale came to the task as a sanitary reformer, at some distance from any organized religious interest. For her, the laws of hygiene represented an order in nature which her class had discovered and which it had a duty to pass on to others. That instruction might be reinforced by small gifts or services but was above all by force of personal example. Thus, the civilized nurse who had absorbed the inner discipline of sanitary living might hope to influence the uncivilized soldiery, either recalling them to their duty or, in her care of their suffering comrades, affirming society's recognition of its obligations. Death in war was not the result of indifferent or ignorant commanders but a part of a higher plan in which each person had an assigned role. That role might be discovered by observation of others and inner revelation but could not be openly taught. In following the prescribed rules of conduct, their meaning would emerge.

Her rivals, like Mary Stanley and the Rev. Mother Bridgeman, leader of one of the groups of Irish nuns, gave these principles an explicitly religious foundation. The will of God was not to be found by personal revelation but through the teachings of His churches. Thus it was important that their patients saw their nurses not just as performers of a social duty but as performers of a *Christian* duty. And, of course, it was important to the nurses that their patients died in an appropriate state of grace. These beliefs tended to give their work a more sectarian character which aroused controversy in a country that was still deeply suspicious of the Roman Church and those thought to be inclined towards it. In some ways, mid-Victorian attitudes to Catholicism were not unlike those to Marxism in our own time. The charge could be used to discredit opponents by implying a lack of patriotism and respect for traditional national values. In fact, the allegations of actual proselytization by the Catholic or High Anglican members of the party are likely to be exaggerated for this very reason. Cardinal Manning was acutely sensitive to the problem and there is ample evidence elsewhere in his work of his attempt to encourage conversion by force of the example set by Catholics in social or public service rather than by direct canvassing. It seems implausible to suppose that he would have deliberately sent a contingent of zealots to the Crimea.

As Summers (1988: 60–5) shows, neither approach could conclusively demonstrate any superiority in the mortality rates of the patients nursed by its adherents. Indeed such improvements as did occur seems to owe as much to the efforts of the Sanitary Commission sent out by the War Office and to the local medical officers as to the nurses. Certainly, the conclusion that the War Office drew was that a permanent, stable corps of medical orderlies was required. Its members would be trained and gain experience which would not be subject to disruption by regimental needs. The female nurses had brought welcomed sympathy and small comforts but their practical contribution was not valued.

The point, however, is again that it was less what people did than the image built around them that was consequential. Florence Nightingale became a symbol which could divert public criticism of the mismanagement of the Crimean campaign by the military commanders. She provided the evidence that her class really did care for the ordinary soldiers dying in droves on this muddy Russian peninsula. But the reality was that most of the caring work continued to be done by the same kinds of people who had always done it: orderlies and soldiers' wives had laboured, head servants had supervised and well-born ladies presided over the whole. What changed was the moral significance of the work. It became dominated by the values of the ladies and they took the credit for it.

The Crimean experience offered a further and more public example than that of the sisterhoods of the ways in which working-class women could be mobilized to impose a new order on their own class. It particularly underlined the need to recruit women without the corrupting experience of industrial employment. At the same time, however, the moralization of nursing defined it as an occupation which could be taken up by women from economically marginal middle-class backgrounds without threatening their social status. Florence Nightingale's character references for the Crimean nurses seeking post-war employment include at least four which seem to be for widowed or orphaned gentlewomen (Summers 1983: 53). The more class boundaries solidified in late Victorian Britain, the more acute became the problem of such women, who lacked the private wealth to sustain their position in society. The widows and daughters of the clergy, the military and the lower strata of the professions needed opportunities to support themselves.

The direct impact of female nurses in the Crimean campaign was limited, if not negligible. But the attention which they attracted gave their most astute self-publicist, Florence Nightingale, an importance as a symbol of progress and enlightenment that profoundly influenced the future development of that occupation. Her programme did not, however, command wide support among those actually charged with the management of the hospitals and the medical care of the sick. The Crimea was a demonstration. Its realization would involve more contention, more compromise and less achievement than Whig traditions in nursing history have allowed.

Chapter four

Making the Myths

When Florence Nightingale returned from the Crimea in 1856 her main preoccupation was with reforming the medical and sanitary regime of the Army. The idea of the Nightingale Fund, its application to nursing reform, and the development of the St Thomas's scheme, discussed in this chapter, were all other people's initiatives. But her talents as a publicist did as much as ever to focus attention on her own contribution and idealizations of nursing. Recent scholarship, has, however, begun to chip away the patina of a hundred years of legend to reveal the complex politics of nursing reform, the limitations of the St Thomas's initiative and the heterogeneous origins of recruits to the occupation. In the process, it obliges us to reappraise the contribution of groups who are often placed on the margin by official historians of nursing, groups as diverse as the pauper nurses of the Poor Law and the VADs of the First World War. This chapter, then, will focus on education and practice from the late 1850s to 1919 in order to examine the social construction of an occupation and its imagery. Its legal construction, from the registration movement of the 1880s through the Nurses Registration Act 1919 to the formative work of the General Nursing Council, forms the topic of Chapter 5.

The Nightingale Fund

The Crimean War had made Florence Nightingale a national heroine. Popular songs were written about her, a cheap biography was produced and her image figured in numerous prints and figurines. There was even a racehorse named after her. At one level she disdained the publicity, refusing, for example, to allow an official portrait to be made for public reproduction. At another she was to use this reputation with skill, ruthlessness and cunning. One immediate result, however, was a flow of gifts and suggestions of a public testimonial. Mrs Samuel Carter Hall, Elizabeth Herbert and the Nightingale family decided to organize this into a national appeal. Provisional arrangements began to be made during August 1855 for a committee to manage the appeal with Samuel Carter Hall and Sidney Herbert as joint secretaries. The first idea was to present something of the 'bracelet and teapot' kind as Parthenope Nightingale described it. Elizabeth Herbert thought, correctly, that Florence would reject this proposal. On further reflection, her friends came up with the notion of funding the establishment of 'an English Kaiserswerth'. This seems to have been put to her in a letter by Sidney Herbert in September 1855, requesting a plan for the use of the Nightingale Fund.

Florence Nightingale remained unenthusiastic but endorsed the general idea of the subscription with reference to some correspondence with Dr Bence Jones. He was an acquaintance from Harley Street days who had written to her in August 1855 asking for her comments on his ideas for the establishment of a nurse training school at St George's Hospital in London. As Cope (1958: 21) points out, there is no evidence that Florence Nightingale had any definite plans for nursing reform before she went to the Crimea. Bence Jones specifically proposed the appointment of a superintendent nurse with the sole duty of teaching and supervising trainees and the establishment of suitable residential accommodation for nurses in training. These were eventually to be distinctive features of the St Thomas's scheme. No reply to Bence Jones survives but further evidence of the seriousness with which his proposal was received can be found in Florence Nightingale's letter to Sidney Herbert of January 1856 recommending him as a member of the council of the Nightingale Fund (Baly 1986: 10–11).

When the fund officially closed in June 1856, £44,039 had been collected 'to establish a permanent institution for the training, sustenance and protection of nurses and to arrange for their proper instruction and employment in hospitals' (Baly 1986: 9). But the fund was not a high priority for Florence Nightingale. Her efforts were focused on getting a Royal Commission appointed to investigate the sanitary management of the Crimean Army and influencing its report. Besides this, she continued to be interested in hospital design. Nursing was a secondary consideration to the physical structure of hospital buildings. Indeed, her writings from this period emphasize the preferability of keeping non-surgical cases out of hospital and of encouraging people to take more care of themselves and their families. Even her famous *Notes on Nursing*, first published in 1859, are directed wholly at home nursing. If she had a vision of professional nursing it was more akin to that of the sanitary missioners which we discuss in Chapter 9.

The fund drifted aimlessly for some time until, early in 1859, Sidney Herbert proposed to use it to support an arrangement between King's College Hospital and St John's House. Florence Nightingale opposed this plan. Baly (1986: 26) suggests that she objected to the religiosity of St John's but this did not prevent her later supporting, with fund money, a midwifery school run at the same hospital by the sisterhood. She also backed the superintendent, Mary Jones, in the dispute over her decision that the nurses should take religious vows. It seems more plausible to accept Smith's (1982: 156–7) view that she was piqued that someone else had taken an initiative.

This interpretation can also be supported by the chronology of developments at St Thomas's. Miss Nightingale had been corresponding with Richard Whitfield, the resident medical officer, since 1856. He had recommended nurses to her and she had referred would-be pupils to him. In 1858, St Thomas's was faced with the need to redevelop its old hospital because of new railway construction that would encroach on the site. Most of the doctors favoured remaining in central London and rebuilding on what was left of the plot but others, including Whitfield, thought that the hospital should be relocated to the suburbs at Blackheath. The court of governors was also divided. Whitfield knew that his preference accorded with the sanitary ideas then being expressed by Florence Nightingale and asked for her support. She mobilized her various social and political connections to this cause.

In March 1859, references suddenly start to appear in their correspondence to plans for the establishment of a nursing school. These seem to have developed without reference to the fund's council. When they were presented to a leading member, the retired surgeon-diplomat Sir John McNeil, he immediately identified their weaknesses, particularly the lack of a suitable superintendent and the restrictive terms proposed for the nurses' contracts which would, he thought, deter recruits. These reservations were shared by at least one other council member, George Bracebridge, who had been in the Crimea with the Nightingale party. Possibly because of these concerns but probably also because Miss Nightingale was much more interested in the architecture than the staffing of the new St Thomas's, the plans made little progress during 1859.

Action appears to have been precipitated by another move from outside Florence Nightingale's control. In December 1859, Mrs Baines, a prominent member of the Ladies Sanitary Association, asked the fund to support their plans for a nurse training scheme, threatening public questions about its management if she were refused. Miss Nightingale brusquely dismissed this threat but there was also immediate action to endorse the arrangements with St Thomas's. It is as if the council were willing to agree to almost anything to be rid of an embarrassment.

Even then a final agreement was not signed until May 1860. This provided for the fund to pay for the board, lodging and wages of each probationer, together with fees to the matron, the resident medical officer, and the ward sisters for teaching. The matron was given absolute authority in the administration of rules devised by Miss Nightingale for the dress, conduct and working, learning and resting hours of the probationers. They were issued with a brown uniform, white cap and apron. Each had her own cubicle in the nurses' accommodation but they were required to pray together twice daily, to eat together and to attend church on Sundays. A monthly discipline return was to be sent to Florence Nightingale. The probationers were required to be single women of good character between the ages of 25 and 35, although young widows and deserted wives seem to have been accepted from an early date. Those who completed the year's training would be obliged to serve for three years in whatever posts they were offered by the executive committee set up by the fund's council to administer the scheme.

Baly (1986: 36–7) makes all the pertinent points about this agreement. Despite Florence Nightingale's strictures, it left the position of the existing staff intact. Mrs Wardroper, the matron, had been left a gentleman's widow at the age of 42 with 4 young children and had to take up employment to support them. She had been appointed matron at St Thomas's in 1853 and remained in that post for thirty-four years. Like most matrons of the period she had been brought in for her experience of household management and made no pretence of being a nurse herself. At the time of the agreement, she had not met Florence Nightingale more than two or three times. Similarly, there was no vetting of the sisters who would give the instruction and there is no evidence of ordinary nurses being displaced. This might not have mattered too much if St Thomas's had been a well-managed and progressive hospital, but it was not. It was, then, unlikely that the new scheme would make any decisive break with the past.

This view is strengthened by Baly's observation that the conditions of service were a 'contract for the servant class'. The provision of uniform clothing and the strict regime of eating, washing and praying are markers of the position of household servants. Nurses would not be in the lowest grades of service:

under-nurses were employed to wash and feed the patients and scrubbers to clean the floors and lay the fires. But they were not expected to be educated women: provision was made to improve their skills in reading and writing. Richard Whitfield was sceptical of their ability to cope with any substantial intellectual material and Flint South, the senior surgeon, and an opponent of the scheme, was on record as considering nurses to be 'in the position of house-maids' who were best taught by experience and example (Woodham-Smith 1950: 275). Sir Joshua Jebb, the fund's chairman, acknowledged in his first public report in 1862 that

> Persons of superior manners and education, ladies in fact are not as a rule required, but rather women of somewhat more ordinary intelligence belonging to classes in which women are habitually employed in earning their own livelihood. (Abel-Smith 1960: 22)

Again, it is the continuity that is more striking than the differences. At its inception the St Thomas's scheme seems to have had no higher ambition than to improve the skills of the doctors' assistants, despite various protestations about creating a new profession for women.

We have looked at these events in some detail because they do bring out very clearly the gap between the mythologies of nursing and the historical record. St Thomas's was not selected as the site of the fund's activities as the result of any process of rational decision making. Indeed, it could even be argued that the nurse training scheme was no more than an inducement to the hospital to accept Florence Nightingale's proposals for its relocation and rebuilding according to her sanitary principles. The first recruits were neither pioneers nor heroines but ordinary women who wanted a respectable way to make a living: 'daughters of small farmers who have been used to household work – and well educated domestic servants' (Abel-Smith 1960: 21–2). This emphasis on recruiting women whose only work experience was in a domestic context suggests at least one lesson had been carried over from the Crimea. Although the agreement between the fund and St Thomas's took a year to conclude, the fitful nature of the correspondence is suggestive of something being hastily organized by busy men and women whose priorities lay elsewhere but who felt obliged to produce some results for their stewardship of publicly subscribed monies.

The St Thomas's experience

Given the circumstances of its origins, it is hardly surprising that the relationship between the fund and St Thomas's began to deteriorate almost immediately. Part of the problem was that the Whitfield–Nightingale factions were defeated over the fate of the hospital. John Simon, then superintendent-general of health at the Privy Council, was determined that St Thomas's should not leave central London and arranged for the offer of a publicly owned site on the Albert Embankment at a favourable price. There were arguments about the design of the probationers' accommodation which would put sleeping quarters in the attics and day-rooms in the basement, impairing the supervision of the nurses off duty.

Florence Nightingale also became disillusioned with Mrs Wardroper and Mr Whitfield. Both had frequent episodes of illness which impaired their control over the hospital. Mrs Wardroper was a woman of limited education, reasonably conscientious but unimaginative. Miss Nightingale, however, appears to have lost confidence in her judgement of staff by the early 1870s and there is evidence of frequent disagreements in their assessment of the character of probationers. There are also suggestions that her life was affected by some personal tragedy in the late 1860s and that this affected her grip on decision making. Mrs Wardroper's relations with Mr Whitfield fluctuated between the amicable and the quarrelsome. Whitfield's lectures to the nurses had been repeatedly criticized for being too orientated towards the medical rather than the nursing care of patients, although it is not clear what was actually meant by this. It is arguable that his critics were actually objecting to his emphasis on a technical rather than a moral approach. Whitfield had also had disputes with the hospital governors in the early 1860s about the legitimacy of his claims for domestic expenses. By the end of the 1860s there was evidence that he was neglecting his contracted duties to the nursing school. He had developed a drink problem and there were hints of a liaison with one of the sisters. The full story seems to have emerged only from a personal investigation by Florence Nightingale in 1872 which was used to force his resignation. Mrs Wardroper continued in office until 1887, when she finally retired at the age of 76.

St Thomas's, however, appreciated the advantages of the probationers as a source of cheap labour and in 1865 proposed an expansion of the school to 45 places. This placed the fund in difficulties since the income from their investments was only sufficient to support about 18 places, and the committee was reluctant to tie up all its resources in this way. The result was a gradual development of special categories of probationer who, either personally or by sponsorship, paid for their own board and lodging and sometimes met their own salary. This also had the effect of broadening the social background of the recruits and producing people who were more obviously qualified for supervising positions in hospitals or infirmaries. No one actually paid for their instruction.

What were the actual achievements of the school? Baly (1986) points out that Mrs Wardroper's records are not always consistent and are difficult to collate. However, she estimates that up to 1871, 188 nurses had been accepted for training, of whom 126 had completed the programme. Of the others, 3 had died, 7 had resigned and 52 had been dismissed, either for misconduct or for ill-health, in about equal proportions. At least 36 of the survivors left nursing within two years. Baly concludes that it is unlikely that there were more than 50 St Thomas's trained nurses at work in hospitals after ten years of the scheme (Baly 1986: 57–61). The wastage rates do not seem to have improved greatly after the move to the new site and staff changes of the 1870s and 1880s. The fund's report for 1900 stated that, since its foundation, 1,645 candidates had been admitted and 982 completed the training. An investigation by the hospital treasurer in 1910 found that 523 candidates had been accepted in the previous seven years, of whom 274 had finished the course. High wastage rates are not a new phenomenon.

The quality of their education was uncertain. The list of duties printed in the school's application form from 1861–1871 sounds comprehensive enough:

Duties of probationer

You are required to be sober, honest, trustful, trustworthy, punctual, quiet and orderly, cleanly and neat.
You are expected to become skillful–
1 In the dressing of blisters, burns, sores, wounds and in applying fomentations, poultices, and minor dressings.
2 In the application of leeches, externally and internally.
3 In the administration of enemas for men and women.
4 In the management of trusses, and appliances in uterine complaints.
5 In the best method of friction to the body and extremities.
6 In the management of helpless patients, i.e. moving, changing, personal cleanliness of, feeding, keeping warm, (or cool), preventing and dressing bed-sores, managing position of, etc.
7 In bandaging, making bandages and rollers, lining of splints, etc.

8 In making the beds of patients, and removal of sheets whilst the patient is in bed.

9 You are required to attend at operations.

10 To be competent to make gruel, arrowroot, egg flip, puddings, drinks for the sick, etc.

11 To understand ventilation, or keeping the ward fresh by night as well as by day; you are to be careful that great cleanliness is observed in all the utensils, those used for the secretions as well as those required for cooking.

12 To make strict observation of the sick in the following particulars:–
The state of secretions, expectoration, pulse, skin, appetite; intelligence, as delirium or stupor; breathing, sleep, state of wounds, eruptions, formation of matter, effect of diet, or of stimulant, and of medicines, etc.

13 And to learn the management of convalescents.

But Rebecca Strong, who trained in 1867, recalled that it was the medical students who took temperatures and pulses and tested urine so that little record-keeping was expected of the nurses. The consultant surgeons inspected the operation wounds and the nurses made poultices but these were actually applied by the dressers. The diaries kept by the nurses for inspection by Florence Nightingale show that most of the probationers' time on the wards was unsupervised and they received little instruction from the sisters. Lecturers commented on the difficulty of teaching a group with such a wide range of ability and previous education. In 1875, for instance, one observed that 'a considerable number of the probationers were not capable of writing with sufficient fluency to keep up with the lecturer' (Baly 1986: 174). The home sister of the time, Mary Crossland, thought the doctors were right to pitch their expectations on the low side, dictating notes, spelling hard words and coining short axioms, although Florence Nightingale reversed her criticisms of Whitfield and started pressing for more advanced scientific instruction.

Perhaps the most telling data, however, are those uncovered by Summers (1988: 92–3) recording the experience of Mrs Deeble and six other nurses, including Rebecca Strong, who had completed the St Thomas's course and then went to work in the Army Hospital at Netley in 1869. In her letters to Florence Nightingale, she reports how, in the first month, one nurse nearly poisoned a patient by giving him liniment rather than cod liver oil. The nurses proved less skilled than the orderlies: they did not know how to administer ether sprays, take temperatures or use glasses to protect patients when applying leeches close to the eye. These orderlies had been trained by the Army Hospital Corps set up in 1857 as the official response to the Crimean experience and its lessons for the care of the sick in the service.

Spreading the message

As in the Crimea, however, it was less the rather uncertain experience at St Thomas's that mattered than the image of its authors. The fund came to be regarded as an authoritative source of advice and guidance by other hospitals, both in the UK and overseas, who wanted to introduce new styles of nursing. Its officers were frequently asked to recommend matrons capable of introducing the new systems. In fact, they were rarely able to do so: only six St Thomas's nurses became superintendents before 1871 and even the loyal Henry Bonham Carter, who was the fund's secretary from 1861 until 1914, acknowledged that only two of these were any good (Baly 1986: 62). Most of the London hospitals took independent initiatives (Rivett 1986: 102–6).

The fund repeatedly emphasized three critical points: that there must be a trained matron with exclusive responsibility for control of the nursing service; that the nurses must be reasonably well paid; and that servants must be employed for the manual labour. The first of these was a sticking point for many hospitals but it was crucial to the Nightingale model, even if it had not been a shining success at St Thomas's. In the past, nurses had been appointed to work on a particular ward. Any training they received was specific to that job and at the discretion of the sister and the doctors. Now the matron was introduced as a third figure who hired the new recruits and organized their formal instruction. Probationers were moved from one ward to another in a pattern determined by the matron. Although the sisters evaluated probationers on their wards, the final judgements were made by the matron and the sisters' reports became a means by which she could also assess their authors. The system attempted to break the fragmented loyalty of the nurses to their wards and substitute a unified allegiance to the occupation and to the moral vision of the class from whom matrons were drawn (Williams 1980, Rivett 1986: 105–11).

This generated considerable opposition from the medical profession. A typical example is the reaction to an article published by Margaret Lonsdale (1880), a nurse at Guy's Hospital, in *The Nineteenth Century*, a monthly magazine. She criticized the doctors' objections to the nursing reforms introduced by a new matron at Guy's in 1879. These included a more formal system of training and regular rotation of sisters and nurses from one ward to another. Miss Lonsdale alleged that the opposition arose from concern that better-educated nurses would identify 'malpractice'. It is not clear what this actually means but the replies from two doctors in the June 1880 issue suggest that they thought it was a criticism of treatment decisions. These responses, from Octavius Sturges of the Westminster Hospital and Seymour Sharkey of St Thomas's, attacked the involvement of ladies in nursing. They were apt to be motivated by self-righteous religious zeal and too ready to challenge medical judgements on the basis of superficial learning. Neither doctor was unsympathetic to the attempt to improve the practical skills of lower-class nurses so that they could administer treatments or monitor the patients' condition more effectively.

> I can see no reason why an educated nurse should not make use of her special senses in the same manner as we do ourselves in order to obtain the same information. . . . I know of nurses who, as I strongly suspect, do actually make use of the stethoscope. I am not going to tell of them, but rather hope that what is now a secret indulgence may be one day among the recognized accomplishments of good nurses. (Sturges 1880: 1094)

Both accepted that there was a place for the lady nurse.

> The duties of a nurse demand as a *sine qua non* physical, those of a sister intellectual power. Ladies are more adapted to supply the latter than the former, more fit to be sisters than nurses in a large hospital. (Sharkey 1880: 1101)

But both saw the issue of control as central.

> (Miss Lonsdale) sneers at the idea of nurses 'studying the character and special requirements and fancies of the particular medical man or surgeon under whom they were placed with a view of gaining his approbation by every means in their power'. But all common-sense people will see that this is a most important part of good nursing, if they allow that its object should be to carry out the orders of the responsible medical officer. . . . However bad the old system of nursing may have been in many ways, and however uneducated and untrained its members, they, the doctors, and the patients regard this benefit, that there was no vaunted antagonism, as there now appears to be, between medicine and nursing. (Sharkey 1880: 1104)

Ladies who wanted to be doctors should take that training: those who did not must learn the discipline of the experienced NCO who saw his subaltern make an unwise decision.

It is easy to ridicule these arguments from a twentieth century perspective. On the other hand, it should be recognized that the doctors' philosophy did represent one possible way of organizing a hospital which had shown itself capable of change and development. The nineteenth century had few models of collegial organization and, even in our time, this has not proved to be an easy way to work in health care settings. There seems no reason to doubt the genuineness of the doctors' belief that their patients' interests would be better served by nurses working under their direction than by a fragmentation of responsibility between themselves and an independent line of nursing accountability.

The issue was further clouded by the contention over the provision of medical education for women. Margaret Lonsdale blurs the boundary between the two occupations when she suggests that women with a medical qualification could combine the functions of doctor and nurse. Dr Elizabeth Blackwell, one of the first women to obtain a medical degree, had been considered as a possible candidate to superintend the King's College Hospital Scheme mooted in 1859 (see p. 40). There was, then, concern that nursing reform might lead to the creation of a back door route into medicine, going in the other direction across this ill-defined frontier.

The doctors' opposition was derived from a belief that women of their own class were constitutionally unsuited to certain forms of education, work and public life. Women were neither physically nor temperamentally equipped to deal with these spheres of human activity. Some women confronted this theory directly, but others turned it back against the doctors. If women were unsuited to medical work, men were unsuited to caring work. If you believed that men and women were endowed, by God or by nature, with essentially different qualities then the whole of social life should be divided between them so that their efforts were wholly complementary. The home might be the main institution where caring work was performed but it was not the only one. Women should do this work wherever it occurred, as in the hospitals, and men should be excluded from it. Florence Nightingale, in particular, was critical of women's attempts to enter male occupations rather than to develop new careers for themselves which could be taken as seriously as those for men. In her view, it was better to be a first-rate nurse than a third-rate woman doctor (Woodham-Smith 1950: 365–6).

While these arguments could be put to hospital governors in promoting the new system, a more significant factor may well have been its economics. Put at its crudest, probationers turned out to be a source of cheap labour for the hospitals, which also discovered that, by improving training and awarding certificates, they could tap a new source of revenue by renting their nurses out for private duty. The development of private work, in particular, was not part of the original St Thomas's scheme.

The voluntary hospitals were under considerable financial pressures by the late 1860s. The costs of treatment were increasing, as were staff costs, both from the recruitment of greater numbers of nurses and from the attempts to improve pay in order to attract a better quality of recruit and to provide new accommodation that would allow her life to be more completely regulated (Maggs 1987: 185–7). One estimate suggests that nursing costs per patient may have quadrupled between 1860 and 1890 (White 1978: 57). These rising expenses led hospitals to consider charging patients for treatment and the principle was widely adopted between 1880 and 1900. St Thomas's was one of the first voluntary hospitals to open a wing for paying patients, in 1881, and Baly (1986: 206) argues that this was a factor in the increasing efforts to recruit 'special' (i.e. middle-class) probationers. The attempt to establish closer control of costs may also have been a factor in the decline of the sisterhoods from the early 1880s onwards, although the loyalty of members to their order must have been a further complication to the disputes over the control of nursing work which hospitals preferred to avoid (Rivett 1986: 109–10).

Hospital governors rapidly came to realize that the introduction of a training school allowed them to reduce staffing costs. As probationers, recruits could be attracted by the promise of training. Indeed, in many hospitals, lady recruits might even be induced to pay for the privilege of being trained. Their fees represented about 2½ per cent of hospital income nationally by 1891, a modest but reliable source of revenue (Abel-Smith 1960: 30). Training periods were gradually lengthened from one to two or three years and the age of recruitment lowered from 25 years to 23 or even 21. Younger women could be paid less and tied to the hospital for a longer period. The success of this policy is noticeable in the way that probationers came to be substituted for ward scrubbers on domestic duties. There is no mention of these at St Thomas's in the 1860s and 1870s but by 1918 the probationers were clearly doing most of the cleaning and polishing (Baly 1986: 209). Maggs (1983: 22–6) shows that the practice was widespread from the 1890s. Moreover nurses could be made to earn a profit. There was a growing demand among the wealthy for nurses trained under the new system which the hospitals realized they could meet by hiring out their own staff. The reputation of the hospital and its training certificate underwrote the quality of the nurses in a way which had not previously been possible. By 1905 the London Hospital was making a profit of £1,700 a year out of the difference between its fees and the costs of both trained staff and probationers (Abel-Smith 1960: 58).[1]

The availability of such a pool of trained labour was an important factor in persuading subscribers to provincial hospitals to contribute towards the initial costs of change. When the governors of the Royal Cornwall Infirmary at Truro introduced the new system of nursing care in 1869, for instance, an important part of the financing was provided by a nursing fund. Subscribers of five guineas could obtain a nurse without further charge, a 2-guinea subscriber had to pay 7/6 a week and non-subscribers paid 15/– a week. The maximum salary for a nurse was 6/8 a week so the hospital should have earned a useful surplus. In fact it did not. Two new head nurses were brought in, trained by Agnes Jones in Liverpool, and the hospital's recruitment advertising began to demand higher educational standards. By 1877, servants were informed that they need not trouble to apply for such posts. But the internal friction caused by these changes, between the head nurses, the housekeeper, and the house surgeon, led to a high staff turnover which hampered the development of the nursing service. Indeed, subscribers were so dissatisfied that a rival private nursing association was set up in 1880. The rows reverberated in this small provincial town and the hospital ran into a considerable financial crisis in the early 1880s. It was only in response to this that the housekeeper was dismissed and her duties taken over by the head nurse in 1882. The title and office of matron passed for the first time from the domestic to the nursing side of the hospital. Nevertheless, the matron remained subordinate to the house surgeon until about 1907 and did not get full control of the nursing and ancillary staff until the 1920s (Andrews 1975: 74–90, 170–1).

The experience of the Royal Cornwall Infirmary should caution us against over-hasty generalizations about the spread of Nightingale-style nursing. Indeed, it is unclear how far that model ever existed outside the mind of Miss Nightingale and her immediate associates. Their writing created a language in which changes could be articulated and legitimized. But the actual form which they took was heavily influenced by the personalities, politics and economics of individual hospitals. It must be remembered, however, that the voluntary hospitals served only a small proportion of the sick. The attention which has been given to them reflects their role in developing the image of nursing as an organized occupation for women. As charitable bodies, they had a vested interest in self-promotion which advanced the reputation of nursing. But if we are to understand the conditions under which most institutional care of the sick was carried out and which led to the state's interest in nursing, we must turn our attention to the Poor Law.

A state nursing service?

As we have shown, Poor Law nursing had already attracted the attention of reformers during the 1840s and 1850s. The physician Dr Edward Sieveking, who was a prominent member of a number of sanitary reform associations, had drafted a specific plan for the training of pauper nurses in 1849 and in 1855 he persuaded the Epidemiological Society to submit a version of it to the Poor Law board, which was the central body regulating the system of poor relief. Women paupers would be trained to act as nurses in the workhouses or for sick people receiving outdoor relief, and could be hired out for private work to the profit of the institution. In the longer term the women would be equipped with skills by which they might earn their own living. The board agreed that the scheme had considerable merits, although it would probably only be practicable to implement it in larger workhouses. A letter was sent to the board's inspectors encouraging them to suggest the idea to local guardians. In fact, however, nothing came of the proposal because of the dearth of able-bodied young women to train and the absence of any workhouse officer capable of instructing them. But it is important to note that much of the opposition came from other reformers such as Dr H. W. Rumsey and Louisa Twining, who felt that the moral character of pauper women was too damaged for them to be able to accomplish the mission of raising the tone of nursing care (Hodgkinson 1967: 559–61).

The situation in the workhouses began to change only after some determined pressure group activity in the early 1860s. There were a number of well-publicized scandals, particularly the death of Timothy Daly at the Holborn Union workhouse in 1864. The editor of the *Lancet*, James Wakley, used this to realize a plan for a private commission to inquire into the conditions in London workhouse infirmaries compared with those in the voluntary hospitals. The results were published in a series of articles during 1865 and 1866 which provide a comprehensive indictment of both premises and organization. Workhouse infirmaries were poorly managed and occupied insanitary and inappropriate accommodation. The commissioners commented on the irony of the way the public and medical profession had 'ignored these *real hospitals of the land*, while lavishing princely munificence on the splendid institutions (voluntary hospitals) which ostensibly supply the national hospital requirements' (Lancet Commission 1866, quoted in Hodgkinson 1967: 472). The pressure was maintained by the formation of an association for improving workhouse infirmaries in February 1866, which brought the *Lancet* group together with the circle around Louisa Twining and the Workhouse Visiting Society. Florence Nightingale was persuaded to overcome some initial reservations and give her support. She had been lobbying the Poor Law board independently since Daly's death in an attempt to obtain an official inquiry. This brought her into contact with the reform-minded Inspector Farnall, who was responsible for visiting London workhouses and became the liaison between the Poor Law board and the association (cf. Rivett 1986: 67–71).

It is important to note this semi-official support. As Hodgkinson (1967: 471) remarks, the *Lancet* investigation received the fullest co-operation from the metropolitan boards of guardians despite the potential implications of its findings. The commissioners were given free access to medical records and to workhouse accounts. Some of this may have been due to a naive expectation by guardians that the inquiry would endorse their economical management and rigorous deterrence of the undeserving. But it seems equally plausible to argue that sections of the Poor Law board and the guardians may have hoped that the publicity would generate pressures for reform which would overcome parliamentary hostility to greater expenditure on the poor. Certainly, Hodgkinson (1967: 487–92) shows that most of the London boards responded quickly to the reports by initiating improvements in their infirmary buildings and appointing additional staff, including nurses. One of these, Matilda Beeton, who worked first at Rotherhithe and then at the Strand workhouses, played an important part in further exposures of filth and corruption which precipitated official investigations for the Poor Law board by Inspector Farnall and its medical officer, Dr Edward Smith, during 1866. Farnall seems to have worked closely with Florence Nightingale over this inquiry and there are suggestions that she may have drafted parts of his report (Baly 1986: 86–7).

The administration of the Poor Law was under particular pressure in 1866 from high cyclical unemployment and a cholera epidemic. Although there was a change of government and a new minister at the Poor Law board, concern had been sufficiently aroused for a broadly bipartisan approach to reform (Rivett 1986: 71–82). In 1867 the management of lunatics and fever cases was centralized under a Metropolitan Asylums Board which also acquired powers to regulate the conditions and appointment of medical officers and the treatment of the sick poor in separate workhouse infirmaries. Similar provisions were made nationally in 1868.

Part of the means of improvement was seen to lie in the introduction of paid and trained nurses. The only existing requirement for this work, prescribed by an order of the Poor Law board in 1847, was the ability to read the labels on a bottle of medicine. Even that, as we saw earlier (p. 12) could not be relied upon. In 1865 the replies by the London workhouses to an inquiry by the Poor Law board showed that they were employing only 69 skilled nurses and 897 paupers. There is no evidence of any provincial workhouse employing a trained nurse before 1863 (Hodgkinson 1967: 562–3). Of course, 'training' cannot be understood in any modern sense at this date. It would have been more like the informal apprenticeship of a domestic servant. Nevertheless, the results of this inquiry and a similar exercise among the provincial workhouses led to circulars in May 1865 from the Poor Law board urging guardians to recognize the responsible nature of nursing work and to discontinue the practice of employing pauper women. Guardians were urged to improve pay and accommodation in order to attract more respectable women to this work.

The first attempt to organize a training programme came in Liverpool in 1865. The administration of the Poor Law in that city had a good reputation for the efficiency and quality of its services. Its infirmary at Brownlow Hill had employed a paid head nurse since 1848 but the actual provision of care was in the hands of able-bodied pauper women who could not be effectively supervised. They were not thought to have the necessary moral qualities to act as reliable assistants to the medical officer or to control the disorderly population of a great port. Although the authorities were aware of their deficiencies, they felt unable to bear the cost of an improved, salaried service. William Rathbone, a local philanthropist who had already initiated a home nursing scheme (see pp. 173–4), offered to fund the introduction of St Thomas's nurses to establish a training scheme for the pauper women. This proposal caused some embarrassment in London: Rathbone wanted 12 trained nurses but the fund probably had no more than 25 available to meet all the requests they were receiving.

It is not entirely clear how many Nightingale Fund nurses ever actually went to Liverpool. Certainly, they had considerable difficulty finding a superintendent. Agnes Jones seems to have been the only candidate available (Smith 1982: 174). Florence Nightingale had considerable reservations about her. She was a committed Evangelical who found it hard to keep nursing and proselytizing separate. Her health was indifferent and she seemed to be weak and easily led by others. Miss Nightingale had opposed her admission to St Thomas's in 1860 and warned Rathbone that she 'lacked the moral authority necessary for his purpose' (Smith 1982: 174). Agnes Jones did not have the complete control of the nursing staff which was prescribed by the fund's usual policies and there are reports of severe conflicts between herself and the workhouse master, the existing staff, and the patients (Smith 1982: 174, Baly 1986: 85, 91).

However, the master gave a generous account of her achievements in a report to the Poor Law Board in 1866 discussing the first year of the scheme (Hodgkinson 1967: 564). He claimed that there had been a marked improvement not only in the state of the wards and the care of the sick but particularly 'in the demeanour of patients on whom the humanizing influence of a body of women of character devotedly discharging their duties, produced evident fruits'. The problem was the dearth of 'women of character': during that year 24 out of 40 probationers had resigned or been dismissed while 83 occupants of the 37 pauper assistant posts had also left in various circumstances. Nevertheless, the authority valued the experiment and extended it from the male wards to the whole infirmary at the ratepayers' expense. The report praised Agnes Jones's contribution and urged the Poor Law Board to support similar developments elsewhere. Dr Edward Smith's report on provincial workhouses in 1867 was slightly more sanguine, suggesting that he had been unable to observe much difference between the two parts of the infirmary but that the medical officers on the male side felt they could place greater trust in their nurses.

Liverpool was not alone in such experiments. Two Protestant sisters with hospital experience had taken over the management of the Chorlton Infirmary during a fever epidemic in 1865 and modernized practice there, despite considerable mortality among their assistants from the disease (Hodgkinson 1967: 565). The Nightingale Fund's work in Liverpool collapsed with the death of Agnes Jones from typhus in 1868. Her death was the occasion for a great eulogy by Florence Nightingale, despite her reluctance to give any support to Miss Jones in her own lifetime. The purple prose of Miss Nightingale's account has clouded any real analysis of Agnes Jones's contribution. There are accounts of her death being accelerated by overwork, rising at 5.15 a.m. and working till 1.00 a.m. the following morning because the infirmary staff would not respond to her direction (Smith 1982: 174). Others see this as evidence of her incapacity to delegate (Baly 1986: 90). But one could ask to whom she could have delegated her tasks. Of the nurses known to have gone from St Thomas's, she had herself dismissed three and two others survived only a few months of their subsequent employment at the Middlesex Hospital before being dismissed as unfit for sisters' posts (Baly 1986: 91). The fund was unable to find a new superintendent for three months. It then sent Louisa Freeman, who only had four months' training at St Thomas's, treated the Liverpool probationers like 'reformed convicts', and resigned within weeks. She was followed by Lucy Kidd who was dismissed in March 1869 by the Liverpool authority for drunkenness, apparently a long-standing problem.

At this point the Liverpool scheme disappears from the traditional histories of nursing. It tends to be depicted as a decision by the fund not to continue its involvement, despite Rathbone's offer of further financial support (Baly 1986: 91–2). However, there are also suggestions that the Liverpool authorities simply drew their own conclusions from the mixed fortunes of the experiment and went their own way despite some vilification from Miss Nightingale for their departure from her doctrines (Smith 1982: 175). Certainly Rathbone was encouraging the Manchester guardians to regard Liverpool as a model when he offered to support workhouse infirmary nurse training there in 1873 (Hodgkinson 1967: 572).

Once again it is hard to resist the conclusion that the Nightingale Fund successfully appropriated the credit for developments which were occurring in many localities throughout the 1860s, while making only a limited contribution of its own. In his 1867 report, Edward Smith observed that there was now a general feeling that skilled paid nurses ought to be appointed and that a considerable number were being engaged by the larger workhouses. The small rural workhouses had been slower to act because they had fewer sick inmates and those tended to be the elderly and infirm who were thought to need less specialized attention. But Smith argued that there should always be a trained nurse supervising the care and that there should be a distinction between domestic and nursing staff, even among the pauper assistants. The combined effect of this report, Smith's earlier report on London and the 1865 circulars gave a considerable boost to the movement away from pauper nursing. It did not eliminate scandals and it did not achieve rapid success but the aspiration to raise standards was firmly established. Progress was much more rapid in the urban areas. In Norfolk, for example, paid trained nurses remained uncommon until the 1890s (Digby 1978: 171).

There were two principal constraints: cost and the difficulty of recruiting trained personnel. The improved accommodation in the new generation of separate infirmaries that were being built or converted from surplus workhouses and the increased use of paid labour raised expenses considerably. Indoor relief, asylum charges for the insane and officers' salaries combined rose from 40 to 70 per cent of expenditure on poor relief between 1862 and 1919 (Crowther 1981: 61). Nevertheless, although salaries, staff accommodation and superannuation benefits improved steadily from the 1860s, they remained inferior to those in the voluntary hospitals until the twentieth century. The nurse–patient ratios were greatly inferior so that the work was heavier. Workhouse infirmaries were not equipped to share in the technical advance of medicine. Interesting acute cases were diverted into the voluntary hospitals while the infirmaries' doors had to be kept open for chronic and incurable patients. Moreover the management of patient services often remained divided between the matron, who was not usually a nurse, and a head nurse. This could be an endemic source of conflict which was not resolved in the nurses' favour until 1913. Finally, the patients continued to be stigmatized as paupers, and subjected to a more rigorous discipline than they would have encountered in the voluntary hospitals. As we have remarked, however, all nursing involves some element of social control so that this is a difference of degree rather than of kind.

Poor Law infirmaries were drawn into the provision of training for much the same reasons as the voluntary hospitals: it lowered costs, stabilized the workforce and helped to expand the pool of appointable personnel. Again, however, this sector lagged behind the voluntary hospitals. The infirmaries had acquired the power to train nurses under the 1867 Act but little use was made of this until the late 1870s. The Nightingale Fund was involved in a successful demonstration scheme at Highgate between 1869 and 1877 but this also terminated in disputes over the control of the staff. Guardians were not willing to abdicate their responsibility for the use of public money to a private trust. In fact, it seems to have been the more stringent approach of the Local Government Board, which replaced the Poor Law Board in 1871, to public expenditure during the economic recession of the 1870s that delayed progress. Momentum was restored only when new private funds were injected through Louisa Twining's Association for Promoting Trained Nursing in Workhouse Infirmaries in 1879 and the subsequent re-entry of the Nightingale Fund to support a programme at St Marylebone from 1881. The association had supported the training of more than 800 nurses by 1898 (Abel-Smith 1964: 45). The Local Government Board gave these developments some official encouragement so that there were 936 probationer nurses in training nationally by 1896 and 2,100 by 1901. But probationers remained difficult to attract, although the minimum age of entry was lowered from 25 in 1873 to 21 in 1900 to give a competitive edge over the voluntary hospitals.

As the supply of nurses increased, the LGB tried to phase out pauper staff. Guardians were forbidden to employ them as nurses after 1887. But the impact of this was not immediately felt, especially in the smaller mixed workhouses in rural areas like Norfolk where the change was to job titles rather than the work paupers were asked to do (Digby 1978: 172). Many such institutions were still not employing trained nurses by 1913 when paupers were finally barred from any employment in sick wards unless supervised by paid staff. The guardians at Banbury, for instance, could not afford the going rate for a trained nurse and were obliged to appoint a woman 'hardly fitted to hold the post of a parlour maid' (Crowther 1981: 180). We shall return to the implications of this judgement.

These problems reflected the reluctance of training schools run by local Poor Law authorities to recruit probationers in excess of their own needs, in the absence of any central subsidy, in order to provide staff for smaller institutions. The same was true of the voluntary hospitals but they were able to make good their deficit by attracting Poor Law-trained staff. There was also a constant leakage into the private sector.

But the concern for the supply of nurses to permit an acceptable standard of care under the Poor Law throughout the country did focus the LGB's attention on the regulation of training to a much greater extent than in the voluntary sector. It must be remembered that there was no nationally recognized examination and certification of general nurses until 1925. Until then, each institution awarded its own certificates, whose value reflected the status of the hospital or infirmary. The witnesses who gave evidence to the Departmental Committee on Nursing the Sick Poor in Workhouses, whose report was published in 1902, were united on the desirability of a national system based on a common syllabus and means of assessment. It was thought that this would help to ease both the absolute and the relative shortage of nurses. The Poor

Law was still struggling with a ratio of one nurse or probationer to every twenty patients while the voluntary hospitals had a one to three staffing ratio (Abel-Smith 1960: 52). A nationally recognized training would increase mobility since its qualifications would be valid anywhere. Greater mobility would be an attraction in itself but would also open more opportunities for promotion which might become more rapid than in the voluntary hospitals. Moreover, it would help to ease the staffing difficulties in the small rural infirmaries. Some witnesses went so far as to call for the establishment of a national Poor Law Nursing Service which would direct women where their labour was needed.

The departmental committee recommended considerable developments in Poor Law nurse training. Two grades of nurse were to be produced: major training schools would give a three-year course leading to a certificate which would allow its holders to be promoted to the higher posts in the infirmaries. Minor training schools would run a one-year course for a less skilled grade of nurse who would be eligible, after experience, to take a shortened course in a major training school to achieve full certification. The committee also wanted to increase the powers of superintendent nurses at the expense of matrons and to require the superintendents to have midwifery training. We shall look at the fate of these recommendations in more detail in the next chapter, but they are important as the first official attempt to open a 'second portal' to nursing.

One of the central themes of Abel-Smith's *A History of the Nursing Profession* (1960) is the struggle between the occupation and its employers for control over entry. On the one hand lay the desire to create 'a new profession for women', an outlet for the moral enthusiasms of Victorian ladies and a respectable alternative to the work of a governess for economically marginal female members of the middle class. On the other lay the managerial and medical view that what the hospitals and infirmaries needed was a large number of skilled hands at the bedside who would be willing to work in poor or rural districts for the wages that local communities or institutions could afford. This is a conflict that recurs and we shall encounter it again when we look at midwifery and nursing outside the hospitals. It is, however, a conflict with important implications for the definition of the occupation and for the social base of its recruitment. Should it be a profession with a high educational requirement which would, implicitly, also mean a narrow class basis for entry or should it be a craft with less emphasis on educational attainment and a broad appeal to women of less exalted backgrounds? Folk histories of nursing emphasize the former and identify Victorian nursing with its aristocratic or plutocratic patrons. We have already commented on its genteel values but it is important to test this image against the actual selection of women to bear those ideals among the poor patients of the hospitals and infirmaries.

Ladies or women: professionals or servants?

As we have shown, nursing was regarded as a superior form of domestic service relying mainly on respectable working-class women until the 1860s. Leadership was provided by what one might call 'distressed gentlewomen', ladies from the middle class who, for some reason, needed to earn their own living and sought to capitalize on their customary skills of domestic management in matron posts. These women would have no background or identity as nurses and the supervision of nursing care was a marginal part of their work. In the orthodox view, the major consequence of the Nightingale reforms was to turn nursing, in the voluntary hospitals at least, into a career for young middle-class women. Although Abel-Smith (1960: 21–2) recognizes the humble origins of the St Thomas's probationers, he argues that they were displaced by a higher class of recruit during the 1880s and 1890s. By 1902, he contrasts them with the recruits to the infirmaries, described by a matron as 'too often of the servant class' (Abel-Smith 1960: 47–8).

In fact it is not at all clear how far this contrast can be sustained. Maggs (1983: 63–88) examined recruitment to two major voluntary hospitals and two large Poor Law infirmaries between 1881 and 1921. He emphasizes that they were all operating in a highly competitive market for 'white blouse' labour. At various times all of them had difficulty in attracting recruits for training and responded by lowering age and educational requirements. Immigrants, from Ireland, Wales, and Scotland, made up about 15 per cent of the recruits. More than 70 per cent of the probationers had some previous work experience. Table 1 shows the distribution of their occupational backgrounds.

What is striking here is the similarity in the pattern of recruitment to these very different institutions. (The variation at Portsmouth is due to the fact that the record series start after the age of recruitment had fallen so that entrants had had less opportunity to acquire an employment history.) The majority of recruits came from domestic service or lower-status areas of nursing like fever or cottage hospitals. Maggs suggests that the 'nil' returns include a substantial number of women who had previously worked in family businesses or farms. The only group of women

Table 1 Distribution of previous work experience of recruits to nurse training 1881–1921 (Based on Maggs 1983)

	Manchester Royal Infirmary (1881–1921)		London Hospital (1881–1921)		Leeds Poor Law Infirmary (1895–1921)		Portsmouth Poor Law Infirmary (1905–21)			
		%		%		%		%		%
Nil	478	28	1240	28	103	28	147	40	1968	29
Nursing	658	39	1161	26	131	35	87	23	2037	30
Domestic service	351	21	1290	29	81	22	42	11	1764	26
Clerical and commercial	66	4	224	5	10	3	28	8	328	5
Clothing and textiles	22	1	84	2	19	5	18	5	143	2
Shopwork	29	2	104	2	16	4	28	8	177	3
Education	85	5	228	5	7	2	3	1	323	5
War work and miscellaneous	7	1	123	3	3	1	14	4	147	2
Totals	1696		4454		370		367		6887	

with any significant education were the teachers and most of those seem to have been uncertificated women who were being excluded from their own occupation by their lack of credentials.

A similar picture is presented by Simnett's (1986) analysis of recruits to St Bartholomew's between 1881 and 1900, although she does show some evidence of gentrification under the influence of Ethel Manson, later Mrs Bedford Fenwick, a leading advocate of the professionalization of nursing. A scheme was introduced for fee-paying 'special' probationers who could attend lectures and work in the hospital for three months, which many better-off young women seem to have used as a trial. Even with this shift towards recruits from professional backgrounds, Simnett points out that a high proportion were orphans who were compelled to earn their own living.

Thus nursing at this period must be seen as a socially mixed occupation which offered respectable employment to domestic servants, office or shop workers and marginal members of the middle classes. It could not have grown on the elitist criteria that some of the ladies would have liked to introduce. The proportion of all women who were in employment did not alter between 1881 and 1911. What did change was their distribution, with a dramatic decline in agricultural and manufacturing work and a corresponding expansion in the service industries. How, then, can we explain the image of nursing as a preferred choice of employment for young women from privileged homes? Part of the answer certainly lies in the high visibility that a few articulate individuals achieved, particularly through the registration movement. But part of it may also be found in the experience of the First World War and the care given to its casualties.

The impact of war

It was extremely unusual for the middle and upper classes to make much use of hospitals during the nineteenth century. This had begun to change from the 1880s onwards with the development of private nursing homes and pay beds in the voluntary hospitals. Initially, these had mostly been intended for members of the middle classes who lived outside London or had no family available to care for them. There was, however, a steady expansion in such facilities. In 1891 there were 9,500 places in nursing and convalescent homes in England and Wales, rising to 13,000 in 1911 and, more sharply, to 40,000 in 1921, of which 26,000 were in nursing homes (Abel-Smith 1964: 189, 339).

This movement had two stimuli. The earliest was the changing nature of medical technology. It was increasingly difficult to meet the requirements of aseptic surgery in a private home and, as early as 1903, the *British Medical Journal* was commenting on the 'growing disinclination' of surgeons to operate under such conditions. Physicians were reaching similar conclusions. Institutional care could provide better supervision of the patient and control of infection than could care at home. These views were further strengthened by the technical advances which occurred during the war, especially in surgery. By 1920, it was no longer possible to contemplate performing surgery anywhere other than an operating theatre, except in wholly extraordinary circumstances.

The second factor was the upper and middle classes' experience of hospital care during the war. It must be stressed that this was atypical. Officers' hospitals, which had been introduced only since the Boer War, had trained nurse to bed ratios as low as one to four whereas the typical military hospital operated with a one to sixteen ratio. For comparison, civilian voluntary hospitals averaged one trained nurse to nineteen beds while the major Poor Law infirmaries had one trained nurse for forty-four beds (Abel-Smith 1960: 85).

The war imposed heavy demands on medical and nursing services. At the outbreak there were about 24,000 doctors for a population of 36 million and about 12,000 nurses with some recognized training. There were about 45,000 beds in 800 voluntary hospitals, another 40,000 in military, fever and smallpox hospitals and about 120,000 in 700 Poor Law institutions. In 1914, it was anticipated that about 50,000 beds would be sufficient for the services' needs. These would be provided by temporary accommodation or by contracting with existing hospitals. By November 1918, 364,133 beds had been made available for military casualties, of which about 318,000 were actually occupied. Poor Law accommodation had been requisitioned on a substantial scale to meet this need (Abel-Smith 1964: 252–3, 281).

Although probationer nurse intakes expanded considerably during the war, the additional nursing input needed to care for these casualties was provided mainly by women of the Voluntary Aid Detachments (VADs) and some smaller independent nursing reserves. These had developed over the previous decade as part of the planning for a major European war. Many of these women had attended some preparatory courses and exercises and most received a three or four month training during the war (Summers 1988). By the end there were 12,000 of them working in military hospitals and 60,000 in auxiliary hospitals, providing service under contract with the War Office. The VADs tended to come from upper- and middle-class backgrounds, partly because many of them were unpaid (only those in the military hospitals received a salary). They posed a considerable threat to the established order of nursing, especially because the patients rarely distinguished between them and the trained nurses. The lady nurses saw the possibility of their exclusive position being diluted while the ordinary nurses saw themselves as likely to be further downgraded by this influx of women from more privileged backgrounds. As a result, there was considerable friction between nurses and VADs, especially in the civilian hospitals.

Vera Brittain records some of this in her memoir of the First World War, much of which she spent as a VAD. She encountered little hostility in the military hospitals, especially overseas, but the civilian hospitals were very different:

> Like other civilian nurses, the Sisters of St Jude's (a pseudonym) hated the necessity of using VADs but I never came across any institution where they showed it so plainly.
>
> Whatever training or experience a Red Cross nurse might have had before going there, they were determined that she should not be permitted to imagine, even for a moment, that this entitled her to any kind of status. The longer a VAD had performed the responsible work that fell to her on active service, the more resolutely her Ward-Sister appeared to relegate her to the most menial and elementary tasks. At St Jude's I was never allowed so much as to attempt the simplest of dressings. I was not permitted even to remember the experience in nursing malaria and pneumonia which I had acquired in Malta and in the medical wards at Etaples. (Brittain 1978: 450–1)

She comments rather ironically on the official report by the Joint War Committee of the British Red Cross and Order of St John, with its claim that, 'The VAD members were not trained nurses; nor were they entrusted with trained nurses' work except on occasions when the emergency was so great that no other option was open' (op. cit. p. 410). The memory it evokes for her, of coming on duty to find her light medical ward had been converted overnight into heavy surgery with forty seriously wounded men straight in from the front line, might be dismissed as a 'great emergency'. However, it is abundantly clear from other points of her story that this was not an isolated occurrence. As an experienced VAD she was regularly taking charge of wards under the loose supervision of a sister who might be responsible for three or four other wards at the same time. This would not just be at

73

night but was a regular day-time practice on both medical and surgical wards. Abel-Smith (1960: 86) quotes Lady Diana Cooper's (1958: 127–8) memoirs of her time as a VAD at Guy's Hospital to note that within a few weeks she was 'giving injections intravenous and saline, preparing for operations, cutting abscesses and once even saying prayers in Sister's absence'.

The link between this hostility and the registration issue was clearly recognized. Vera Brittain contrasts the willingness of the military hospital in Malta to give lectures on nursing to VADs with the reluctance of the First London General (a military annexe to St Bartholomew's Hospital situated in Camberwell) to provide instruction 'chiefly, so I always imagined, because they were afraid of VADs getting to know too much'.

> This . . . attitude to VADs was typical of the nursing profession as a whole, especially in England, where the introduction of semi-trained Red Cross probationers into military hospitals had pushed to a crisis the thirty-year-old struggle for the registration of nurses. The Matron at Camberwell was always scrupulously just to us in practice, but we must have been bogies to her in theory, for she and other promoters of state registration evidently visualised a post-war professional chaos in which hundreds of experienced VADs would undercut and supplant the fully qualified nurses. Actually, this fear was groundless; all but a very few VADs were only too thankful when the War was over to quit a singularly backward profession for their own occupations and interests, but many 'trained women' having no such interests themselves could not believe that others were attracted by them. The presence of Red Cross nurses drove some of them almost frantic with jealousy and suspicion, which grew in intensity as the VADs increased in competence.
> (Brittain 1978: 309)

If the VADs gave the nurses a common enemy against whom they could unite, these volunteers nevertheless played their part in the revolution in public attitudes brought about by the experience of wartime medical care. The officer classes came to see that institutional care need not mean the squalor of a Poor Law infirmary or the doubtful company of social inferiors in a voluntary hospital, but could involve recovery in pleasant surroundings associating with one's equals and cared for by competent and personable young women of one's own class.

By the end of the First World War, the organizational context of general hospital nursing had changed considerably. There had been great developments in medical technology which made new demands on nurses. The social mix of patients was being transformed by the influx of middle-class people to the private wings of voluntary hospitals. Nursing was increasingly being constituted as a separate department of both voluntary and Poor Law institutions with its own line of accountability to the governing body. As an occupation it had received the limited recognition of an official category in the censuses since 1861 (Davies 1980). But its identity remained ill-defined and bitterly contested.

The social background of recruits had changed much less than might have been imagined since the 1830s. Although a handful of well-born women had become matrons or lady-superintendents, the majority of those describing themselves as nurses still came from relatively humble backgrounds. They were better educated than their predecessors but, of course, elementary schooling had been compulsory for everyone since the Education Act 1870. They had experienced the very different social discipline of the late nineteenth century. This was particularly marked by the decline of the sisterhoods and the secularization of the hospitals. An explicitly religious basis for control was no longer relevant. Nevertheless, as Maggs (1983) emphasizes, they were mostly ordinary women who needed to earn their living.

This division was of considerable importance in the struggle to organize nursing more formally as an occupation both in defining its boundaries and in establishing its status within the division of labour. Was nursing to be a 'new profession for women' with a graduate entry and parity of esteem with medicine? Or was it essentially a refined form of domestic service, drawing on the formidable skills of many servants but assigned a clearly subordinate place in the hospital? Was 'proper work for nurses' the management of servants or carrying out the hands-on services themselves? Given the changing nature of the patient population there was a further problem in establishing the 'correct' relationship between patients and nurses. The incorporation of the handywoman class had defined nurses as the controllers of poor patients. The arrival of the middle classes in hospital called this into question. Should the model evolve towards that of the private duty nurse, the servant of the patient? Could this be reconciled with the very different missions of Poor Law and voluntary hospitals, the former still marked by the spirit of moral reform while the other slid into the amorality of commerce? Would employers be willing to match the aspirations of the most ambitious nurses or would they be compelled by the economics of care to resist the pressures for gentrification?

The principal arena for contests over the resolution of these questions was the struggle for registration which began in the 1880s and is still in many respects open. The next two chapters will focus on this issue and the arguments over whether nurses should be registered, so that the occupation would be closed to all but those with particular credentials, and who should control registration and, hence, define what was and was not to be counted as nurse education and nursing work.

Chapter five

The Search for Unity

Claiming membership of an official occupation involves something more than checking a box on a census form. That act does represent a process of self-definition, of identification as an engineer rather than a production manager, a director of a small company rather than a jobbing plumber, or a part-time nurse rather than a housewife. At the same time, it is a claim to belong to a group whose boundaries are socially rather than individually defined. To represent oneself as a member of an occupation is to assert that one should be included in a category of people who share some distinctive skill.

> An occupation consists in part in the implied or explicit *licence* that some people claim and are given to carry out certain activities rather different from those of other people and to do so in exchange for money, goods or services. (Hughes 1971: 287)

The idea of a licence is more than just a metaphor. In modern societies all occupations are, in a sense, defined by law. At its most basic, anyone claiming the status of an occupation member is under a legal duty to perform their work to the standard of competence that can reasonably be expected of any member of that group. Failure to do so may be the basis for a claim of negligence, whether the task is mending radios or giving injections.

In some occupations, however, the process of claiming membership is formalized by a legally backed system of credentialling. Legitimate claimants are identified by their possession of specific certificates which confer the right to use the occupation's title. For example, only people with qualifications recognized by the General Dental Council may legally describe themselves as 'dentists', 'dental surgeons', or 'dental practitioners'. In a few cases, it is actually made illegal for anyone who does not hold a particular credential to perform certain tasks. Only registered medical practitioners, registered midwives, and student members of those occupations can lawfully deliver babies, for instance.

As Freidson (1986: 63–91) shows, credentialling is not associated in any simple way with the social standing of an occupation, although members often see it as an important symbol in claims to the status of a profession. Its wider significance is as an element in the demarcation of the occupation's boundaries and the discrimination of 'insiders' from 'outsiders'. In the later part of the nineteenth century, nursing was a heterogeneous occupation. The title 'nurse' was still applied to a wide variety of people from very different backgrounds performing a range of tasks and holding a great diversity of qualifications. Many of these had little currency beyond the institution which had issued them. Credentialling, in the form of registration, would bring some order to this chaos. The pressure group activity associated with the registration debate has been described in detail by Abel-Smith (1960). Our interest here lies more in the sort of order which the various parties wanted to impose and in analysing their success or failure.

The registration movement

The debate over nurse registration was essentially a struggle between those who wished to maintain the supremacy of the organizational interests of the hospital and those who wanted to reconstruct nursing as a free profession which controlled its own fees and conditions of work. Each faction hoped to use training and the credentials awarded on completion to institutionalize its own preferred version of nursing. The conflict revolved around a complex mixture of economic interests and gender rivalries. These are most clearly set out in the various parties' evidence to the Parliamentary Select Committee on Registration which reported in 1904. Up to the end of the First World War, however, the whole issue was largely regarded with scepticism, indifference or bemusement by the political audience whose support would be required for the legal imposition of credentialling in the form of registration.

The campaign for registration found its most articulate leader in Ethel Gordon Manson (Mrs Bedford Fenwick). She was the daughter of a wealthy Scottish farmer and step-daughter of an MP. From 1881 to 1887 she was matron at St Bartholomew's Hospital in London, resigning on her marriage to Dr Bedford Fenwick, a leading medical politician. Apart from nursing reform, she was also an active campaigner for women's suffrage (Hector 1973).

Her connections and enthusiasms combined in a view of nursing as a high status occupation for women, whose organization and economic relations with patients would be comparable to those of medicine. This model was most nearly realized in private duty nursing and its individual contractual relationships with patients and their families.

Mrs Bedford Fenwick's unyielding views on the autonomy of nursing made her both a formidable protagonist and an uncomfortable colleague. She split from the Nurses' Section of the British Hospitals Association in 1887 to form the British Nurses Association (BNA). When this received a Royal Charter in 1893, she resigned because the new constitution involved an increase of medical influence and deprived her of personal control. Her next move was to form the Matrons' Council of Great Britain and Ireland in 1894 and, in 1902, the Society for the State Registration of Nurses as vehicles for her radical version of the cause.

Private duty nursing represented the largest proportion of the nursing labour market: around 70 per cent in the years up to 1914 (Maggs 1983: 131). Its growth was, however, hampered by the nature of hospital training, the influence of the voluntary hospitals over the supply of private staff, and the difficulties of indicating differences in the quality of the services being offered.

At the end of the nineteenth century, nurse training was tightly linked to the specific work of particular hospitals. Nurses learnt practical skills which reflected the predilections or prejudices of individual doctors or ward sisters. Such knowledge was not readily transferable to other types of patient or to other institutional contexts. The registrationists proposed that this should give way to a 'general' or, more accurately, a 'generalizable' training that would enable nurses to handle a wider range of patients both inside and outside hospitals. It was argued that this would be more efficient since one general nurse would be able to deal with, say, both medical and surgical aspects of a patient's condition rather than two specialists being required (HMSO 1904: 3). Such a development would require a more advanced technical training in the common principles of nursing. In effect, it introduced a medical model for nursing education with a foundation in medicine, surgery and obstetrics prior to any subsequent specialization.

The supply of private nurses was also distorted by the activities of the voluntary hospitals. Amy Hughes, superintendent of the County Nurses Association, claimed that 29 out of the 58 general hospitals in England and Wales had private nursing staff available for hire (HMSO 1904: 79). This partly reflected the difficulty of signalling the quality of care offered to prospective employers. In the absence of nationally recognized credentials, one obvious way to guarantee the standard of service was to trade on the reputation of the supplying hospital. One alternative was to set up agencies or co-operatives which might also establish organizational reputations for quality. The best of these operated on a commission of 5–7½ per cent of a nurse's earnings. The worst might take 25 or even 40 per cent (Abel-Smith 1960: 58). But agencies were subject to what they regarded as unfair competition from the voluntary hospitals' use of student labour, which, as we showed earlier (p. 60), had become a significant source of revenue by the early 1900s. Both, however, were equally vulnerable to undercutting by the least scrupulous agencies which made no pretence, except perhaps to clients, of employing trained nurses at all.

Similar problems affected the development of nursing homes, which we discussed earlier. They were an extraordinarily diverse set of institutions. Some were owned by doctors, others by lay people. Some offered only medical treatment, while others were fully equipped for surgery. Some were primarily for convalescents and others offered active and doubtful forms of physical therapy or massage! Those catering for incurables and the chronic sick were said to have particularly low standards of care (Abel-Smith 1964: 84). But a few of the nurse-owned homes represented themselves as self-conscious alternatives to the lay-controlled voluntary hospitals with care directed by professional nurses and doctors attending only as consultants. Some offered training (Abel-Smith 1960: 111).

Their interest in obtaining a form of regulation that could be used to eliminate competitors coincided with the more general concern of the registrationists to establish employer-independent credentials for nurses. In a sense, the nursing home was seen as the institutional alternative to private duty work. Thus three of the early registration bills placed before parliament combined controls over the training and qualifications of nurses with provisions for the licensing of nursing homes.

These developments were seen as significant threats by the voluntary hospitals and by sections of the medical profession. Both groups recognized that such changes would have an adverse effect on their economic interests and would destabilize the existing division of labour and gender order in health care.

In the absence of a national system of credentials for nurses, the voluntary hospitals had created what were essentially a series of captive labour markets. The job-specific nature of training produced a class of skilled assistants who depended upon that particular hospital for employment. In the absence of transferable knowledge, nurses could not easily move to other institutions. This restricted the scope for either hospitals or nurses to force up wages by competitive bidding or migration from one employer to another. Labour costs to the hospital were further reduced by the widespread practice of shedding staff as soon as they were trained and might expect to earn a skilled worker's rate for the job. Moreover, as we saw above, the hire of private nurses made a useful addition to the hospitals' income.

If the hospitals allowed the occupation to organize itself and create a more homogeneous market, they recognized that their influence would be matched by that of a monopolistic supplier of nursing labour. Instead of nurses working on terms set by the hospitals, the hospitals would have to employ nurses on terms set by the occupation. Hospital governors and administrators foresaw significant rises in wage costs. In 1902, each trained nurse cost a hospital about £57 per year in salary and other expenses, while a private nurse might cost her employer £80–100 per year on the same basis (Abel-Smith 1960: 55). The latter would generally work shorter hours on lighter duties. If the suggestion of treating probationers as supernumerary were adopted, the cost of staffing an average ward would more than double (Maggs 1983: 121).[1] More generally, the hospitals feared that their staff turnover would rise, imposing extra costs in recruitment and induction, and that labour discipline would be weakened.

The position of the Poor Law authorities is less clear. They had been considering the question of a national system of credentials and training for some years and Scotland had actually had a scheme in operation since 1885 (Maggs 1981). White (1978: 117–18) argues, however, that the Local Government Board was put off the idea by its experience of midwifery registration and the way that this seemed to have been used by voluntary interests to attack Poor Law services. She also quotes an attack from the *Poor Law Officers Journal* on the 1906 attempt to promote a bill.

> At present there is going on a gradual appreciation of the value of Poor Law nursing and the services of nurses trained under Poor Law.. . . But as the National Poor Law Officers' Association point out, if this Bill were allowed to go through Parliament there would be nothing to prevent the proposed Central Nursing Board from declining to recognize Poor Law infirmaries as Training Schools under the Bill, or from so framing their regulations as to make it impracticable for the great majority of Poor Law infirmaries to qualify as Training Schools. *We know what has already happened in regard to the Central Midwives Board.* (Emphasis added)

We shall review the effects of the Midwives Act 1902 in Chapter 8.

Members of the medical profession were divided in their reaction to proposals for registration. Elite practitioners were mostly either indifferent or supportive, reasoning that developments in nursing were unlikely to have much effect on the institutions where they worked or the class of patients whom they treated. Many general practitioners were seriously concerned, though. Registration revived their fears over the potential competition from professional nurses, especially for simple cases in rural areas. We shall examine the basis of these anxieties in more detail when we discuss district nursing and midwifery, but the GPs' opposition was forcefully represented by the Incorporated Medical Practitioners Association to the Select Committee on Registration (HMSO 1905: 82).

As is typical in such debates, everyone claimed to be representing the best interests of the patient. The registrationists argued that a register would guarantee that the paying public would be treated only by highly educated nurses of proven technical competence and reliable moral character. An extension of training and the abolition of salaries for probationers would have the effect of producing a closed occupation recruiting mainly from the middle classes.

There is, however, surprisingly little evidence of public or medical dissatisfaction with the technical competence of the 'trained' private nurses then available. Any complaints seem to have been confined to those nurses dealing with the growing numbers of acute treatments in hospitals (Abel-Smith 1964: 102). It is, of course, arguable that patients and doctors are not the best judges of nursing care, but the contrast with the volume of complaints about mid-nineteenth century nursing is striking. Even if the registrationist programme had been fully implemented, it is clear that much of it was irrelevant to the actual needs of private patients. Most of the demand was for the care of the chronically sick (HMSO 1904: 84). The voluntary hospitals were, by now, mainly centres for acute treatments. Indeed, the nurses with the most relevant experience were probably those in the Poor Law hospitals who were largely ignored by the various active protagonists.

Most of the debate, then, focused on the moral character of the nurse. Indeed, as one contemporary commentator remarked, 'to be a private nurse is a severe test of character' (Tooley 1906: 263). The hospital spokesmen depicted nursing as a practical craft whose successful execution depended more on personal characteristics than intellectual skill. The Hon. Sydney Holland (Lord Knutsford), chairman of the London Hospital governors, considered nursing to be 'so childishly simple, you cannot invent a difficult [examination]' (HMSO 1904: 55). Dr Norman Moore from St Bartholomew's Hospital declared that book learning was of little value to the nurse (HMSO 1904: 49).

This anti-academic bias inverted the value structure of medicine where intellectual achievement was highly prized. The opponents of registration were continuing to express the 'separate' spheres theory of the complementarity of men and women as bearers of different qualities in social life. A doctor would be engaged for his skill, a nurse for her virtue (HMSO 1904: Appendix 2). The registrationist case asserted a consistency of values where moral and technical qualities were of equal importance and shared between men and women alike (HMSO 1904: 7). Thus their challenge was not merely to the particular relations between doctors and nurses but to the whole theoretical foundations of the gender order in health care.

Their opponents responded to this indirectly by emphasizing the subordinate status of nursing. Registered nurses would have inflated views of their position, 'expect too much' and be unwilling to undertake dirty or domestic tasks (HMSO 1904: 56). As Sydney Holland bluntly remarked, 'we want to stop nurses thinking they are anything more than they are, namely the faithful carriers-out of the doctor's orders' (HMSO 1904: 37). In this respect they seem to have been better judges of the public mood than the registrationists. It is certainly not difficult to find complaints from employers of private nurses about them 'getting above themselves' (e.g. Donnison 1977: 141). As we show later, there was also a real concern that lady nurses would be reluctant to care for the poor, providing the domestic support necessary in working-class homes, when a woman was incapacitated by sickness or childbirth, at a fee the family could afford.

Although friendly back-benchers regularly introduced private member's bills for registration, the government refused to give them any special priority or support. The nurses' case was hampered by the divisions in their own ranks between the extremists of the Bedford Fenwick faction and those who were more willing to compromise with hospital and medical interests. These cracks were papered over by the formation of a Central Committee for the State Registration of Nurses in 1908 but the occupation was never sufficiently united to put consistent pressure on legislators. It was faced by powerful lobbies in the voluntary hospitals and the medical profession and lacked either the sponsorship of a government department or overwhelming public endorsement of its aims.

Government intervention

With the outbreak of the First World War, the procedure for introducing private member's bills was suspended and the debate about registration moved out of the public arena. Historians of nursing have traditionally explained the eventual introduction of a government bill at the end of the war as the combined outcome of the occupation's unity in the face of potential dilution from an influx of VADs and a movement of public and political sympathy towards measures which enhanced the status of women, reflected in the extension of the franchise in 1918. A closer examination of the record, however, suggests that the reasons may have been more complex and that registration was, paradoxically, a significant defeat for the registrationists.

It is indisputable that the war had had a considerable effect on public attitudes towards women in general and nurses in particular. As we have just shown, it had been difficult for pre-war employers of nurses to conceive of them other than as high-grade domestic servants whose professional aspirations were out of keeping with their social status. Now, even the cynics conceded that women had to be taken more seriously. As Lord Russell remarked with less tact than candour:

> The position is this, women now have the vote, they have to be considered more than they used to be. It is not so easy to say 'I don't like this registration of nurses'. Women are now likely to get what they insist on having. . . . (Earl Russell: *House of Lords Debates*, 27 May 1919, col. 846)

Statements like this would seem to vindicate the Bedford Fenwick strategy of linking registration with suffragism. On the other hand, it is also clear that both the voluntary hospitals and the government had shifted their ground. We must, then, examine registration in the context of the political and administrative reconstruction of Britain after the war. What were the various objectives of the hospital governors, the civil servants and the politicians which combined to produce a government bill for registration in 1919?

Although some die-hards among the voluntary hospital governors continued to resist registration to the bitter end, the expansion of medical services in the First World War and the administrative chaos produced by the lack of any standard system of credentialling had persuaded most that some such scheme was now unavoidable (Abel-Smith 1960: 87–92). The flood of volunteers, coupled with the redistribution of nurses between hospitals and sectors and the return of former nurses to employment, had stretched the capacity of administrators to achieve an appropriate structure for the grading of staff and the matching of skills and needs. In response to this, several prominent voluntary hospital figures who were playing leading roles in the co-ordination of wartime medical and nursing services approached the major training schools with a proposal for a College of Nursing. This would operate a system of voluntary accreditation, ensuring a basic uniformity of curriculum and assessment between the various training schools, whose successful probationers would then be entered on the college's register. Such an approach was far more attractive to the hospitals because it left them with considerable influence over the standards required. The Bedford Fenwick group, which had taken control of the Central Committee for the State Registration of Nurses, continued to advocate the imposition of occupationally determined standards, regardless of their practical implications.

When the private member's procedure for legislation resumed at the end of the war, each faction hastened to present its own registration bill to parliament, in May/June 1919. As Abel-Smith (1960: 94-5) shows, the rival bills were carefully constructed to give an appearance of equity while enshrining their sponsors' control of the registration body. Consequently, while each bill attracted a measure of support, each also aroused sufficient opposition to prevent any real progress.

It was at this point that the government took a hand. Dr Christopher Addison, who was presiding over the reorganization of the Local Government Board into the Ministry of Health, attempted to mediate between the two factions. He stressed, however, that the government was committed to the principle of legislation and was only prepared to respond to the occupation's rival leaders to the extent that they were willing to reach a swift agreement within certain limits. The government's motives, as is usual in such matters, were a mixture of organizational and humanitarian considerations.

The Ministry of Health was created in June 1919 as part of the government's plans for reconstruction. Although it did not initially assume many new functions, its amalgamation of the responsibilities of several other departments with those of the Local Government Board and the National Insurance Commission gave it a central role in the government's social programme. This was intended both to inspire the ordinary soldier in the promise of a 'land fit for heroes' and, later, to contain the social unrest caused by the disruptive effects of the war on the national economy. As the war ended, the Lloyd George administration was stirred by the threat of industrial disorder, particularly in the cities of the north and in Scotland, and by the apparent influence of revolutionary ideals from Russia. Lloyd George himself went so far as to characterize the clashes between police and strikers in Glasgow as 'Bolshevik risings' (Morgan 1979: 48). The Ministry of Health was held out as part of a package of social reform which might contain such pressures on the existing order.

From an administrative point of view, it was essential that the new department should be able to identify a workforce capable of delivering the new service efficiently. Registration was one method by which this might be accomplished. 'Efficient' nurses could be recognized and helped to move freely to the places where they could best be used. At the same time, the administrators seem to have been concerned to ensure that their control of the Poor Law sector was not diluted. The LGB's experience with the Central Midwives Board appears to have functioned as a negative lesson in this respect (cf. White 1976). The Board's 'cavalier' approach to the approval of Poor Law institutions as training schools was criticized in the report of the Departmental Committee set up in 1909 to examine the operation of the Midwives Act 1902.[2] But the politicians also appear to have been worried about the reliability of this labour force.

The war had given an important boost to the organization of women workers by trade unions. In line with the general trend towards increased unionization of the workforce, female membership of unions had risen from 183,000 in 1910 to 1,086,000 by the end of 1918 (Drake 1920: 111).[3] Trade union activity among nurses was not widespread and was confined mainly to the Poor Law and mental nursing sectors. Nursing activists, however, recognized the sensitivity of the government and hastened to adopt some of the language of unionization (*Brit.J.Nursing* 1919: 237). A Professional Union of Trained Nurses was formed in 1919 to recruit general and private duty nurses, promising the use of trade union strategies for professional ends and attacking the College of Nursing as an 'employers' combine'.[4]

Registration was presented as a possible answer to this challenge. In one of her editorials Mrs Bedford Fenwick proposed that it would have a 'pacifying effect':

> The passing of a Registration Bill will do much to allay nursing unrest, and organisation throughout the nursing world will follow. (*Brit.J.Nursing*: 29 March 1919)

'Organisation' here seems to be contrasted with the disorganization that would result if events were left to take their course. It is both a promise and a prophecy.

The message was heard in parliament. Lord Ampthill, for example, used it as an argument in the House of Lords debate on the College of Nursing Bill. If there were delay,

> you will force nurses into trade unions. It is what is already happening. You have seen it in the case of the Asylum Workers' Association[5] and you will force nurses to form trade unions in order to secure what they regard and rightly regard as a right to them, you will simply throw them into the arms of the Labour Party. Is that a desirable thing to do at the present time? (Lord Ampthill, House of Lords, 27 May 1919)

Registration, then, could be both a way of removing a grievance that provided scope for industrial agitation and of bringing greater order to a confused situation, order not only in the sense of definition but also in the sense of discipline.

As Lord Ampthill hinted, however, there were other interests involved. The Labour Party had made an issue of the poor wages and conditions offered to nurses by the voluntary hospitals. They were not alone in this: Dr Addison had frequently expressed his concern and returned to it in the debates on registration:

> I am sorry to say that the payments which have been made to nurses have often been of a discreditable kind, in my opinion much less than the wages of an ordinary cook or kitchen maid. (*Brit.J.Nursing* 1919: 329)

Although the Labour Party had accepted the redefinition of the occupation as a skilled craft, looking forward to the elimination of 'sweated labour in the noble profession of nursing' (*Brit.J.Nursing* 27 September 1919: 182), there was concern that it should not become socially exclusive. The Bedford Fenwick Central Committee Bill was criticized in the House of Commons by Josiah Wedgwood, who became Chancellor of the Duchy of Lancaster in the first Labour Government in 1924.

> We have got to see that the avenue into the nursing profession is kept open for the daughters of the working classes as much as any other class. I observe that we are putting the whole future of the nursing profession outside the control of Parliament . . . I am not at all certain in this handing over to a body which must necessarily become to a certain extent at least, an aristocratic and autocratic body. Quite naturally they desire to keep the profession preserved to those particular people and their

friends. (*House of Commons Debates*, 28 March 1919, quoted by Abel-Smith 1960: 95–6)

In the event, these were probably less influential than the organizational concerns but they provided additional force to the government's general inclinations.

Conferences were arranged between representatives of the Ministry of Health, the Central Committee for State Registration, the Association of Hospital Matrons, and the College of Nursing.[6] The nursing organizations were swiftly disabused of any notion that the government intended to allow them to reconstitute the occupation as a free profession with the independence of medicine or the law. Dr Addison had assured his cabinet colleagues that the bill would be 'confined within the smallest possible compass' and that it would merely set up a suitably composed council which would work out detailed regulations (Ministry of Health 1919: PRO.MH55/462). But all these regulations would remain subject to approval by the Minister. In addition, he would have the power to hear appeals against council decisions to deny accreditation to training schools and to oversee the council's finances. The nurses would have to meet the costs of registration but the ministry was determined to deny the council sufficient resources to permit independent action. Moreover, the occupation was not given any protection from competition comparable to that afforded to midwives by the Midwives Act 1902 (see p. 158). Although the title 'Registered Nurse' was protected, there was no power to make this a pre-condition of employment. Nor did the council establish a monopoly of nurse training. The Royal Medico-Psychological Association, for instance, continued to play an important role in the examination and certification of mental nurses until 1951 (Nolan 1986: 21). Technically, then, the General Nursing Council is more accurately described as a certifying than a licensing body. To the extent that registration did become a pre-condition of employment, this was as a result of decisions by employers taken in the light of the requirements of specific tasks and their ability to recruit people to perform them.

The minister also assumed the power to nominate the members of the caretaker General Nursing Council. It was here the extent of the original registrationists' defeat first became apparent. The council was made up of 9 lay members and 16 nurses. The nursing membership was dominated by the College of Nursing and, with the support of the lay members, they had a comfortable majority of 19 votes against the 6 which the Bedford Fenwick faction could rely on (Abel-Smith 1960: 102).

One marked feature of the nominations was the lack of Poor Law representation. Only 1 of the nurse members had a Poor Law training and 2 out of 6 matrons ran Poor Law hospitals. It is conceivable that the minister expected to safeguard their interests through his power to approve the council's actions. However, the department may also have anticipated that participation in the council would give Poor Law nurses expensive ideas about possible improvements in their training facilities. Given the more active union organization in the public sector, the pressures might have been more difficult to resist. The limited participation of Poor Law nurses would be consistent with the ministry's desire to retain control over that sector.

But the activities of the council can also be seen as a way of extending government influence over the voluntary hospitals, which were subject to review at the same time by the newly constituted Consultative Council on Medical and Allied Services under Lord Dawson and the Cave Committee on the financing of the sector.[7] The war had imposed financial stresses on the voluntary hospitals from which they never fully recovered and which eventually played an important part in their nationalization in 1948. Even at this point senior civil servants like Sir Robert Morant, the first permanent secretary at the Ministry of Health, were considering ways in which public subsidy could be used to achieve more co-ordination with the Poor Law, as it had been in the absorption of voluntary schools by local education authorities since the Education Act 1902. The minister's powers over the GNC would make it possible to use this as another instrument in that enterprise.

The caretaker council

The founding members of the GNC faced a formidable task. They were required to devise a set of rules which would define who could be admitted to the register and would be eligible to vote in the elections for future councils. In so doing, they could, for the first time, impose a common identity on this heterogeneous group of women and men. As the various factions had seen, this would allow the council to have a significant hand in shaping the future course of the occupation's development.

But part of the heterogeneity derived from the sheer diversity of the health care system itself. It was estimated that there were about 1,500 training 'schools' for nurses in 1919. This made the council's task very different from that of the General Medical Council which was required to oversee medical education in only

24 centres. Moreover, the place of student nurses in the economy of both Poor Law and voluntary sectors was so firmly established that any proposals by the council which significantly altered the contribution of students to the hospital workforce or, indeed, made a hospital unable to employ them at all had consequences for the availability of health care which could not be ignored by national planners.

The Bedford Fenwick group fought a determined rearguard action in defence of its vision of a rigorous training modelled on that of the medical profession, with its pattern of a general foundation followed by specialization, and indifferent to the staffing needs of particular institutions. But the early years of the GNC were marked by the institutionalization of a regime which gave a much higher priority to the development of a wide dispersion of improved skills and to the encouragement of local arrangements to rationalize training provision. On the few occasions when the council did attempt to take a stronger line, it was rapidly brought to heel by the ministry or by parliament. The two most conspicuous examples of these conflicts are those over the supplementary registers and over the imposition of a common curriculum on nursing schools.

The supplementary registers

One of the first priorities of the caretaker council was to produce a statement of its educational policy objectives. This seemed to promise a broad generalist approach to nurse training. It should direct the mind to a 'wider outlook than that obtained within the four walls of an institution' and ensure that 'curative measures would be brought into line with the no less important branches of preventive work' (*Nursing Times* 7 May 1921: 498). This aspiration, as we have seen, goes back to the original mission of nineteenth century nursing for the reconstruction of social discipline on hygienic principles. In reality, it had always been compromised by the demand of the hospitals and the medical profession for a skilled subordinate class of labour.

This compromise was reflected in the provision of the Nurses Registration Act for the maintenance of supplementary registers, in addition to that for general nurses. This proposal was completely anathema to the Bedford Fenwick group, which attached great importance to the notion of a common entry route for all nurses. Isabel McDonald, secretary of the Royal British Nurses Association, commented that:

If you are going to establish a supplementary register for fever nurses, perhaps one for children's nurses, it may be for health nurses, perhaps nurses trained in sanatoria, then . . . you can have if you like, nurses for the Zoological Gardens. (*Hospital* 1 February 1919: 389)

The so-called specialists were disparaged as semi-educated and unduly susceptible to medical domination, an objection which went back to Mrs Bedford Fenwick's original opposition to the separate licensing of midwives. This attack, however, also paralleled the medical profession's disdain for groups like lithotomists, whose specialist activities were not founded on a generalist training. What Mrs Bedford Fenwick was opposing was not the medical model of professional organization but medical intervention in the government of nursing.

The caretaker council, however, were under pressure to produce a scheme of registration which would embrace all types of nurse. It had, with difficulty, agreed by November 1921 on an initial criterion of one year's training in an approved hospital. But the actual vetting of applications was left to a sub-committee chaired by Mrs Bedford Fenwick. She obstructed progress on the determination of eligibility to such effect that the majority of members of the council submitted their resignations, leaving it inquorate. They were only persuaded to withdraw by an assurance of ministerial support and the threat that he would amend the Act if disruption continued.

The defeat of Mrs Bedford Fenwick in the first council election in 1923 removed her obstruction. The new council, however, remained determined to proceed on terms which would have had the effect of barring admission to the register to many *bona fide* (i.e. experienced but not trained in a recognized institution) nurses and all VADs. The register was due to close in July 1923 and the ministry indicated its concern about the scope of its exclusions in a letter of March 1923. The council proposed a rule amendment which continued to deny entry to VADs but gave some flexibility on the admission of *bona fide* nurses. Despite heavy lobbying by the council and the main nursing organizations, this change was itself amended in parliament to permit a considerably more liberal approach (Abel-Smith 1960: 103–12). The sponsor of this further amendment, Dr Chapple, explained his thinking in an interview with *Nursing Times*:

if the Nursing Council had made a reasonable rule that met the case, if they had interpreted the Act properly, we should not have touched the matter at all. We did not want to interfere. But the Act has not been properly interpreted. The Council and the College [of Nursing] misled the nurses; to act as they did, to be narrow and to refuse to play fair is the thing that degrades the profession, and not the admission of *bona fide* workers. To refuse a good nurse because she trained in a nursing home or a special hospital, never dreaming she would be under a disability, was cruel and inconsistent. (*Nursing Times* 28 July 1923: 716 quoted by Abel-Smith 1960: 111)

The council were, then, forced to adopt an approach to registration which accepted the persistence of a heterogeneous and segmented occupation.

This was welcomed by groups like sick children's nurses who feared that exclusion from the register would pose problems in the recruitment of members and hoped to gain status from their association with general nursing. Others, however, like the male nurses working in mental asylums, were extremely reluctant to be absorbed. We shall examine the history of this group in more detail in Chapter 7, but they had been able to obtain a nationally recognized certificate since 1891 under the auspices of the Medico-Psychological Association, which brought together the medical superintendents of the asylums. Although this was a voluntary body, its influence was such that possession of the certificate had become more or less essential for advancement in mental nursing.

The MPA had expected to obtain delegated powers under the Nurses Registration Act to continue with its established system of training and examination (*Nursing Times* 7 May 1921: 504). The GNC, however, were reluctant to hand over any powers to a medically controlled body and set out to substitute their own examination and certificate, the RMN. The combination of union hostility to 'general hospital snobs', who represented a possible source of cheap female labour, and the support of the medical superintendents, preserved the MPA certificate as the main qualification in this sector throughout the inter-war period (Nolan 1986: 21–2).

The GNC ultimately recognized four supplementary registers, covering sick children's nurses, mental nurses, male nurses and fever nurses.[8] However, its constitution enshrined a bias against these segments of the occupation by allocating only 5 places to them out of 16 nursing seats on the council, despite the very large number of registrable staff working in the mental sector. Its actual ability to discriminate was limited, though. External pressure had prevented the council from adopting even the moderately exclusive line of the anti-Bedford Fenwick majority. The survival of the supplementary registers was too important to employers as a way of restricting mobility out of the less attractive areas of nursing work. Even then, these areas were able to compete for recruits only by lowering the age of entry and the educational standards demanded, relative to general nursing.

A common core?

The GNC did make some attempt to impose a unified foundation on the various special branches of the occupation. All nurses would be required to sit a common preliminary examination. This was intended to set a minimum national standard which would increase mobility and accelerate training for other parts of the register. In fact, it tended to devalue the supplementary trainings by implying that 'general' training was the necessary prerequisite for all nursing. This was reinforced by the tendency of employers to demand multiple qualifications for promotion in the supplementary areas, although this may also have had an economic basis in that it obliged nurses to work for longer periods on probationer rates of pay. It certainly had the effect of further obstructing the movement of staff out of these specialties and underlining the greater prestige of a general qualification.

But, while these informal effects of the council's actions were of considerable practical importance to ordinary nurses, their formal powers remained severely limited. The definition of educational standards proved contentious, for instance. Here, the problem lay in the diversity of the institutions offering training to nurses. Whatever was proposed had to be acceptable to hospitals varying greatly in size, wealth and patient mix. A first draft for a common syllabus was drawn up by Alicia Lloyd-Still and Marion Agnes Gullen, matron and sister tutor respectively at St Thomas's.

Their proposals reflected the resources available to a large voluntary hospital dealing with a fairly selective group of probationers. They were immediately criticized as unworkable in smaller institutions whose recruits had less education. Miss Cummins, matron of the Liverpool Royal Infirmary, commented (*Nursing Times* 7 May 1921: 502) that, while it might be desirable to raise the present standard, the GNC should 'not lose sight of the fact that moral and not theoretical qualifications went to make the nurse'. On the other hand, Miss Barton, president of the Poor Law Matrons' Association and matron of Chelsea Infirmary, welcomed the proposals (*Nursing Times* 7 May 1921: 503), considering that nurses should be taught to think and how to wish to learn. This reaction suggests that the ministry's concern that registration would raise the expectations of Poor Law nurses had some basis in reality.

Once again, though, the council ran into parliamentary trouble. The smaller hospitals were able to lobby backbench MPs and the ministry, pointing out the problems that these proposals would create for them in recruitment and training costs. The ministry rejected three proposals from the GNC for the approval of a compulsory syllabus, a stand which was endorsed by the Parliamentary Select Committee which investigated the council in 1925. The Select Committee declared its reluctance to do anything which might aggravate the problems of small hospitals 'in supplying an adequate training in competition with the larger and better equipped hospitals [so that] their supply of nurses, already short, might tend to be further reduced' (Abel-Smith 1960: 112–13), Eventually, the council had to settle for a voluntary syllabus.

An alternative option would have been to use the council's powers of inspection and approval of individual schools as a means of imposing common standards. The GNC proposed a number of schemes for the grouping of small hospitals for training purposes. These would have allowed students to obtain more diverse clinical experience and for the groups to support a more extensive educational staff. In practice, however, the voluntary hospitals remained too jealous of their independence to collaborate in such schemes and the council's resources were too limited to press them. There was no budget for a full-time inspectorate and much of the accreditation was based on postal questionnaires completed by the schools themselves. Nor did the council have the effective powers over the public hospitals that would have been necessary to push through a comprehensive rationalization of the system.

Several attempts were made to withdraw accreditation from small voluntary hospitals as a means of encouraging a more co-ordinated approach. When the Nurses Registration Act was being drafted, the ministry had anticipated that this was likely to prove a controversial matter and provided for appeals to the minister from council decisions. While this might have been intended by Morant and his colleagues as a means of achieving a positive influence over the planning of the system, it operated, in the different political and economic climate of the 1920s, as an important brake on the council. Loss of accreditation could impose a financial burden on a hospital that would tip it into insolvency. The ministry was not prepared to see local services jeopardized by the actions of a body with a narrow responsibility for education. Moreover, any move against a particular hospital was likely to stir up strong backbench opposition from local MPs in the House of Commons, as in the case of proposals to withdraw recognition from hospitals in Durham in 1925 and Hastings in 1927. In the unstable political circumstances of the 1920s, ministers were inherently unlikely to risk such a confrontation over what was, in national terms, a fairly trivial matter.

The ministry had never been prepared to concede even this possible degree of influence over the public sector. The GNC was not given any power to inspect Poor Law hospitals, which were subject to review by the ministry's own staff. The council railed against this from time to time, criticizing the ministry's inspections as perfunctory and sporadic. The ministry remained unmoved: it would not relinquish its own powers, because its responsibilities ran more widely than just assessing training provision, and dual inspection would be wasteful at a time of great pressure on public expenditure.

Conflicts over inspection continued throughout the inter-war period. The council kept pressing for authority to appoint full-time inspectors and being obstructed by the ministry, although its income from fees and investments would have made this possible without resort to public money. By 1935, for instance, the council had accumulated a surplus of £80,000 in liquid assets which it proposed to use for this purpose. The ministry suggested that this surplus would be better employed in reducing registration fees! Eventually, in 1938, the council decided to proceed on its own initiative with the appointment of two full-time inspectors, paid out of investment income. This move was, however, overtaken by the outbreak of war, which imposed the need for co-operation between the occupation and the state.

The GNC: a study in failure?

Thus far, relatively little work has been done by historians on the internal operations of the GNC beyond the Whig version presented by Bendall and Raybould (1969). Even Abel-Smith (1960) relies largely on accounts in the nursing press, much of which had a more explicitly sectarian character at that time, and on the published reports of various committees inquiring into the council or its stewardship of nursing education. It is, then, difficult to draw firm conclusions about the relations between nursing organizations, the GNC, and the Ministry, and the pressures which shaped the development of the occupation.

Nevertheless, it seems reasonable to argue that the inter-war years saw the comprehensive defeat of the elitist Bedford Fenwick model for the future of nursing. The criteria for admission to the register were kept open and the training schools left largely untouched. The common preliminary examination was a shadow of the registrationist proposal for a medical model of curriculum organization. Some gains were made in requiring certification as a precondition of certain types of public sector employment but, as we show later, in our discussions of midwifery and community nursing, where these requirements were introduced, the effects should not be exaggerated. The widespread rejection of the council's writ by the mental nurses was a serious block on any aspirations to create a more unified occupation. By 1939, nursing was certainly somewhat more homogeneous in terms of recruitment, skills and training than it had been in 1919, but one must still be cautious in assuming that it had the sort of coherence that it acquired in the post-war period. Registered nurses might share a common certificate but could have gained this out of a great variety of clinical and educational experiences.

Probably the most important changes that had occurred had been demographic. As Abel-Smith (1960: 118–24) shows, the average age of recruits had been falling and the spread of living in had discouraged married women from taking up or practising the occupation. The older widows or deserted wives who had formed a significant component of the handywoman element in the nineteenth century had been largely eased out by the late 1930s. One consequence of this had been a persistent perception of a shortage of nurses. Indeed, as Abel-Smith stresses, this is crucial to the analysis of policy developments during the inter-war period.

Registration had occurred at the only point in the twentieth century when, thanks to the influx of VADs, there appeared to be a surplus of nurses which could provide a basis for a more selective occupation. No sooner had this been accomplished than the surplus evaporated. Some of this was attributable to shorter working hours and genuine expansion in demand. But much of it clearly resulted from the attempts of the GNC to impose an unrealistic entrance standard. Abel-Smith (1960: 154) points out that the effect of demanding secondary education to the age of 18 from all entrants would have involved recruiting almost every single girl who left school at that age during the late 1930s. This would, for example, have left virtually none to train for school-teaching, let alone the office employment which continued to expand throughout this period.

In effect, then, the handywoman class was excluded from the developing occupation rather than from the hospitals. Abel-Smith (1960: 155–60) underlines the expansion in the employment of ward orderlies and uncertificated nurses during the 1930s. Local authorities began to develop training programmes for assistant nurses, especially in hospitals for the chronic sick. This move was strongly resisted by the nursing organizations, although the GNC seems to have been more willing to entertain the idea of some sort of second-tier qualification.

The GNC was set up at a very particular historical moment when many social and economic changes seemed possible; hopes which were rapidly dashed by the post-war economic crisis and the continuing depression of the 1920s and 1930s. Although the effects of this should not be overstated, it imposed a considerable reluctance to embark on social programmes which would introduce large new expenditure commitments. Any aspiration towards the absorption of voluntary hospitals into a nationally planned system which might have been entertained by Morant and Addison disappeared with the former's premature death and the latter's fall from office in 1921. Thus the GNC lost any role it might have played in setting a standard which would have pushed the voluntary sector towards accepting state funding rather than bankruptcy. Indeed, the modest recovery of voluntary hospital finances as the result of the spread of insurance schemes among employed workers in the early 1920s decreased the incentive for co-operation.

The experience of the GNC in the years before the Second World War is notable mainly for its illustration of the limits on the occupation's autonomy. With the possible exception of the socio-demographic shift, which may well owe more to the capture of the recruitment process in individual hospitals or local authorities by particular segments of the occupation, the GNC effectively found itself unable to make any move which imposed greater costs on training schools, whatever its merits from the perspective of the occupation. Just as in the nineteenth century, the economics of health care proved more potent than the ideals of the nursing leadership.

Chapter six

The Nationalization of Nursing

The introduction of registration and the educational policies of the
GNC failed to unify the occupation because they left the existing
divisions in the health care system unaltered. Once the confusion
of the First World War had dissipated, the voluntary and public
sectors went their own ways. Their managers could see no
particular gains to be made from change and the civil service did
not expect the conditions of wartime to recur. The protectionist
employment strategies of the pre-war period were revived, to
discourage the free movement of nurses and the consequent
pressure on wage rates. Now they even had a statutory backing in
the compartmentalization of the nursing workforce by the supplementary registers. While this had strengthened the hand of general
nurses in defining their work and concerns as the core of the
occupation, the continuing fragmentation of the register and the
proliferation of employers perpetuated foci for alternative occupational identities among other groups of nurses. These divisions
were reflected in the sheer variety of trade unions and professional
associations which attempted to organize nurses during the 1930s.
It was only with the imposition of order on the health care system
under the renewed stress of wartime that any more homogeneous
definition of nursing was established.

Drifting through the 1930s

The policy initiatives of the 1930s demonstrate the lack of state
interest. There was widespread dissatisfaction over pay, conditions
of service and standards of education which were seen to combine
in depressing recruitment and encouraging industrial militancy by
nurses. But the remedies proposed by the various factions within
the system were vulnerable either to the limited perspective of
their advocates or to the combined weight of their opponents. No

one group had the power to promote positive changes but many had sufficient to veto them. Nevertheless, three broad strategies can be identified, linked to hospital managements, to the trade unions and to the College of Nursing.

The hospital managements' position can best be seen in the report of the *Lancet* Commission. This was a private initiative launched in December 1930 by the medical journal, on the model of its great investigations in the nineteenth century (see pp. 61–2). Its terms of reference were to:

> inquire into the reasons for the shortage of candidates trained and untrained, for nursing the sick in general and special hospitals throughout the country and to offer recommendations for making the service more attractive to women suitable for this necessary work. (*Lancet* 1932: Preface)

The voluntary hospitals were strongly represented among the commission's membership and it included only two nurses, both matrons. Its analysis and recommendations are heavily influenced by the special circumstances of the voluntary sector.

The shortage of recruits was linked to an alleged decline in the attractiveness of nursing as a career for well-educated and, hence almost inevitably middle-class, girls. Nursing was thought to be losing out to business, social work and teaching as a 'suitable' form of employment for such women. No statistical evidence was produced in the report to justify this and, as we showed in Chapter 4 (pp. 69–71), it is unlikely that the occupation ever did recruit substantially from this class. In 1939, the Athlone Committee was to demonstrate that the main competition for recruits was then coming from low-level white collar posts in the commercial sector – clerks, typists and shop assistants (Ministry of Health 1939: 22).

Given this assumption, and the financial insecurity of the voluntary hospitals, the main emphasis of the *Lancet* Report's recommendations lies on non-monetary changes in the conditions of nurses. This type of recruit was not thought likely to be motivated purely by financial considerations and was expected to have sufficient family resources to be independent of her income from employment. At the same time, she was considered likely to chafe at the restrictive discipline devised for Victorian servants with compulsory attendance at meals, regulated bedtimes, a system of late passes and fines for staying out and a rigid hierarchy of social relationships between staff. By the 1930s, it is not clear that parents would have demanded such restrictions as the price of allowing their daughters to live away from home. In her autobiographical account of training at the Westminster Hospital, for example, Doreen Swinburne (1941: 72–80, 151–2), who was by no means unsympathetic to the need for an element of discipline, contrasts the harshness of the hospital regime with the experience of her own home: returning late after a car breakdown was greeted with amusement by her father and outrage by the sister at the nurses' home. Survival involved developing a host of petty strategies for evading rules. Those who failed or could not tolerate the dishonesties left the occupation. The reform of such regimes would have been relatively inexpensive but there were considerable vested interests in their survival. Many of the practices criticized by the *Lancet* Commission endured long enough to be attacked by the National Board for Prices and Incomes investigation in 1968 (NBPI 1968).

The *Lancet* Commission strategy was not unattractive to the College of Nursing which saw itself as the representative of the occupational leadership. Full membership was confined to registered general nurses, excluding student nurses, nurses who were qualified for only one of the supplementary registers, and assistant nurses. The college consistently emphasized policies which drew the sharpest possible line between their members and others employed in nursing. They shared the social aspirations of the *Lancet* commissioners, which they thought could be advanced by keeping payment during training low enough to discourage all but those girls who came from families with private means. But the interests represented by the commission would not necessarily have gone on to accept the college's corollary, that the occupation could then be reconstructed as a 'proper middle-class profession'. Equally, it is not clear that the college membership would have been entirely sympathetic to the liberalization of student conditions proposed by the commission. The college, understandably, also placed more emphasis on the importance of appropriate financial rewards for career nurses, from whom it drew its support. Both groups, however, spoke for only a minority, albeit an influential one, of nurses and hospitals. Their lobbying efforts were matched by the very different approach of the trade union movement to which both were equally opposed.

Hospitals had been excluded from most of the statutes which had been passed during the nineteenth and early twentieth centuries to regulate the hours and conditions of industrial workers. As a result their pay, working environment, and terms of employment were determined largely by the play of market forces and whatever degree of industrial organization nurses had been able to establish in the face of hostile employers. The difficulties of organizing led the relevant union interests to place considerable emphasis on legislative change. The National Asylum Workers Union had tried to get a statutory restriction on the working week in 1920, during discussions on the possibility of legislation to impose a general 48-hour limit. This had been unsuccessful, but Fenner Brockway, a backbench Labour MP, tried again with a private member's bill in 1930. This would have established a maximum 44-hour week, at a time when the average was in excess of 56 hours, and imposed higher pay rates, especially for probationers. Brockway's initiative did not attract support from the College of Nursing, who had not been consulted in advance. The whole idea of external regulation was attacked as 'unprofessional' and the erosion of differentials between qualified staff and students was seen as a fundamental threat to a major plank of college policy. The voluntary hospitals were appalled by the cost implications and the proposal found no government support. Presumably, the ministry recognized that it would also have substantial implications for public expenditure at a time of deepening economic crisis. Fenner Brockway lost his seat in the 1931 general election and this particular proposal was extinguished (Abel-Smith 1960: 138-9).

It is however an important marker of the interest of the labour movement in the position of nurses, interest which was rapidly fanned by the *Lancet* Commission Report. Although the unions disagreed with many of its proposals, they were quick to recognize its value as an exposé of hospital conditions and its implications for the staff barred from college membership. As in 1919, a socially exclusive occupation would cut off an important career for young women from the respectable unionized working class. Most of the major general and white-collar unions attempted to recruit nurses at some point in the 1930s. They met with substantial success among Poor Law and Public Health Department staff where there was already more of a tradition of union activity and, arguably, greater recruitment from family backgrounds favourably disposed to membership. For the most part, this recruitment was not in direct competition with the College of Nursing, although certainly in opposition to its policies.

The major exception was NALGO (National Association of Local Government Officers) which was not then affiliated to the TUC. They had a number of local government nurses in membership and sought an agreement with the College of Nursing on the formation of a national joint committee to negotiate pay and conditions for this group. This was the subject of discussions with the Ministry of Health, and a related approach by the college seeking a ministry inquiry into the supply and demand for trained nurses, in 1935. Neither of these moves came to anything and they may be best seen as spoiling devices intended to recapture the initiative from the increased activity of TUC-affiliated unions.

This activity, however, was less effective than it might have been because of the fragmentation of effort. Unions were in competition with each other as well as with the college. Eventually, in 1937, the TUC formed a National Advisory Committee for the Nursing Profession to co-ordinate efforts. This issued a Nurses' Charter, which combined traditional trade union proposals such as fully transferable superannuation arrangements and the establishment of Whitley Council machinery for the national negotiation of pay and conditions of service with demands for educational improvements at both pre-and post-registration levels. These moves captured the attention of national news media. Newspapers carried extensive coverage of internal criticisms of the circumstances under which nurses had to work. The campaign was sustained by well-organized demonstrations such as the Guild of Nurses' march down the Strand in opposition to the 'spread-over' (split-shift) system of duty operated by the London County Council. The guild was a branch of NUCO (National Union of County Officers) which also persuaded the TUC to organize parliamentary sponsorship for another Limitation of Hours Bill to reduce the nurses' working week to 48 hours.

The College of Nursing sought to discredit the media coverage of the TUC initiative, calling its criticisms of established conditions 'hostile and unreliable' and attacking the bill as 'impractical' and inappropriate for professionals. The Ministry of Health, however, was concerned by the weight of public support for the well-documented grievances of nurses, by the growth of industrial militancy and by the parliamentary pressure for a policy response to the Limitation of Hours Bill. A renewed approach by the college for an inquiry offered a means of buying time for the situation to calm down. The result was a committee under the chairmanship of the Earl of Athlone, set up in 1937 to:

> inquire into the arrangements at present in operation with regard to the recruitment, training and registration and terms and conditions of service of persons engaged in nursing the sick and to report whether any changes in those arrangements or any other measures are expedient for the purpose of maintaining an adequate service both for institutional and domiciliary nursing. (Ministry of Health 1939: 4)

These are probably the most comprehensive terms of reference that any inquiry into nursing has ever been given and it is probably unfortunate that the committee's work was aborted by the outbreak of war. Its interim report has a clarity of analysis shared by few other official documents on nursing. Apart from scotching the notion that the occupation really was competing in a mainly middle-class labour market, the committee established that the nursing shortage had very little to do with the supply of recruits and everything to do with the continuing growth in demand. By 1939, the voluntary hospitals were employing three times as many nurses as they had been at the beginning of the century. The Society of Medical Officers of Health estimated that there had been a 52 per cent increase in the nursing staff of local authorities between 1928 and 1938 (Webster 1985: 5; Ferguson and Fitzgerald 1954: 286–97). The growing sophistication of medicine and its concentration in hospitals required more care-taking staff than traditional methods of recruitment could provide. The Athlone Committee recommendations were designed to restore its competitive position in the labour market and closely reflect those of the TUC Charter, including a 96-hour fortnight, universal and transferable superannuation provisions and national negotiating machinery on pay and conditions.

The cost of implementing these proposals would clearly be substantial. This prospect was particularly unwelcome to the voluntary hospitals whose financial position was deteriorating again after its brief stabilization in the 1920s. National salary scales and superannuation arrangements would oblige them to match the higher standards of the municipal hospitals without the latter's access to public funds. In London alone, it was estimated that the implementation of the Athlone recommendations would cost £200,000 per year (Webster 1985: 5). As the British Hospitals Association, which represented this sector, acknowledged, such increases in expenditure would push many institutions into bankruptcy.

The outbreak of war provided a convenient excuse for inaction on the Athlone Report. At the same time it also precipitated the staffing crisis which everyone had seen as inevitable and compelled government intervention to impose a solution.

The government intervenes – again

Although there had been repeated calls during the inter-war period for closer co-operation between the public and voluntary hospitals, it was only the demands of wartime which, as in 1914–18, imposed a coherent pattern on the system. The Emergency Medical Service required all designated hospitals, irrespective of their status, to receive casualties. They were brought into a regional scheme of planning and staffed by full-time salaried medical officers. In return, the voluntary hospitals were given exchequer subsidies, which rapidly became an indispensable source of income. The government also found it necessary to embark on a substantial programme of re-equipment and capital investment to make good the deficiencies revealed by the completion of the first official survey of hospital provision in 1941.

The attempt to construct an integrated national hospital service had an inevitable impact on nursing. Planning was originally based on an estimate of 1–3 million casualties from air raids requiring 34–67,000 trained nurses to provide care (Ferguson and Fitzgerald 1954: 296). They would be supported by a Civil Nursing Reserve, comprising women with previous training and experience and untrained volunteers to be known as 'nursing auxiliaries'. The government did not, however, take any immediate steps to offer concrete incentives to recruitment, relying on general appeals to patriotism. One important discovery from the surveys of provision, though, impelled action. This was the extent to which the problems of nursing supply were not just of quantity and quality but also of distribution. If the ministry were to direct nurses to the hospitals where they were needed and to establish a proper relationship between the payments to the nationally organized Civil Reserve and regular hospital staff, national pay scales were essential (Webster 1985: 6). In April 1941, the government imposed standard rates somewhat in excess of those previously offered by the municipal hospitals and substantially more generous than those in the voluntary sector. The financial implications further deepened the government's involvement in sustaining the running costs of the hospital service.

This was intended as only a temporary measure pending the establishment of a longer term method of determining nurses' pay. In fact, such machinery proved difficult to establish because of the sectional jealousies between the various organizations representing nurses. Although most of them supported the idea in principle, each hoped to use it as a way of disadvantaging their rivals. The result was predictable: the government imposed its own solution in the form of a committee chaired by Lord Rushcliffe in October 1941 and modelled closely on the recommendations of the Athlone Report. This gradually broadened its terms of reference to cover conditions of service as well as salary determination. It was comprised of an employers' panel and an employees' panel. Paradoxically, considering its long-standing opposition to state involvement in nurses' pay negotiations, the Royal College of

Nursing was allocated more seats on the staff side than any other individual organization. This was an important precedent, since the Rushcliffe arrangements were perpetuated almost unchanged in the NHS Whitley Council, despite the disputes between the various staff side groups over the relationship between seats and actual membership figures.

The Rushcliffe Committee produced its first report in 1943, recommending substantial increases for trained female staff in line with the RCN policy of widening differentials between registered and unregistered employees. The report was rapidly accepted and implemented but had a minimal effect on the supply of nurses. By focusing its incentives on those who were already qualified, it was, by definition, doing nothing to attract women into the occupation. The drawing power of other types of war work may underline further the extent to which nursing was really in competition with skilled manual or white-collar work for women. The committee's approach actually intensified the problems of distribution. Nurses and hospitals colluded to evade attempts to direct staff where they were thought to be needed. The overestimation of air raid casualties had led to acute shortages in civilian hospitals for TB and other chronic diseases, for the mentally ill and for maternity cases, but most of these were institutions which had little to attract staff. National scales abolished the pay differentials that had been one aid to recruitment.

The problem was alleviated to any degree only when the Control of Engagement Order covering women aged between 18 and 40 was applied to nursing in September 1943. In effect, this meant the conscription of nurses. Unless they were undertaking further training, nurses could leave their current appointment only for one on a priority list maintained by the Appointments Offices of the Ministry of Labour. The loophole exempting further training was widely exploited to evade the regulations, to the benefit of maternity hospitals offering midwifery courses but to the continuing detriment of other shortage areas.[1] Eventually, in April 1944, the ministry took the power to direct newly qualified nurses away from their training schools to relieve shortages elsewhere. The 'further training' exemption remained, however, with the result that 91 per cent of newly qualified nurses elected to go on to other courses rather than allowing their employment to be directed by the ministry (Abel-Smith 1960: 178). The Ministry of Labour continued, rather anomalously, to retain the responsibility for nurse recruitment campaigns until 1957.

The experience of wartime health services had two important consequences for nursing. One was the acceptance by all political parties that there could not be a return to the pre-war heterogeneity of health care provision. Many of the emergency arrangements were likely to become permanent institutions in the post-war welfare state. As a result nursing would take place within a more uniform framework of planning and administration that would reduce the structural bases for internal diversity and conflict. The second, which partly resulted from the same attempts to create a more coherent pattern of provision, was the attention given to the place of nursing within a division of labour. This was less fully developed in the immediate post-war period but its core question – which tasks need to be performed by qualified nurses and which could be done by less skilled and less expensive staff – has remained an enduring concern.

The nationalization of health care

As in the First World War, the demands made on citizens prompted consideration of the sort of society which should be constructed after the hostilities ended. Health and social services were inevitably part of this process of review. In June 1941, Sir William Beveridge, a Liberal economist, was appointed to chair an inter-departmental committee on Social Insurance and Allied Services. This produced a report in 1942 proposing a comprehensive scheme of social security, which assumed that there would be matching access to health care. The Committee on Reconstruction Priorities accepted this and advised the War Cabinet to plan for a comprehensive health service covering all forms of preventive and curative treatment. This recommendation was endorsed by the cabinet and officially announced in February 1943 (Webster 1988: 57–9). There was, however, little unanimity within the government on the form the service should take and only the sketchiest of plans were discussed inside the Ministry of Health before the end of the war.

The formation of the National Health Service has been discussed at length elsewhere and we shall not review it in detail here.[2] The key point is to recognize how much of the previous structure was actually left intact. In many respects, the foundation of the NHS was no different from the measures of industrial nationalization under the 1945–51 Labour Government in that existing personnel and organizations were left largely intact. While the ownership of the assets and the sources of revenue and capital changed, the culture of the institution was preserved. Since 1911, the health services had been organized in a tripartite fashion: independent voluntary hospitals; general practitioner and supplementary medical services administered by the insurance panels set up under the National Insurance Act 1911; and a miscellaneous collection of public health and poor law services which all came under local authority control in 1929. The National Health Service Act 1946, which came into effect in July 1948, perpetuated these distinctions and made little contribution to the development of an effectively planned and integrated service, although, of course, the removal of cost barriers to access was of great practical importance to ordinary people.

The only genuine administrative innovations came in the hospital sector where the voluntary and municipal hospitals were merged. Three tiers of administration were constructed: below the ministry came 14 Regional Hospital Boards and 377 Hospital Management Committees. But the picture was again complicated by the concessions to traditional interests. As part of the minister's strategy for dividing the medical profession and overcoming the BMA opposition to the NHS, 36 teaching hospitals were given an independent status, with their own Boards of Governors reporting directly to him.

The 1946 Act did not specify the constitution of either RHBs or HMCs beyond providing that the minister should consult local universities involved in medical training, local authorities, and such other bodies as he thought appropriate. There is little evidence of pressure from nursing organizations for consultation on this, or indeed any other aspect of early NHS legislation or policy. In fact there was considerable opposition to appointing people in any sort of representative capacity. The TUC questioned this in 1946 and was firmly informed of the minister's view that these

> bodies shall consist of members appointed for individual
> suitability and experience, and not as representatives or
> delegates of particular, and possibly conflicting interests. This
> means that members of RHBs and HMCs could not be
> appointed to 'represent' the health workers. . . . The difficulty
> here would be to draw any line which would keep membership
> of the Boards and Committees down to reasonable numbers. If
> the nurses were to be consulted, why not also the hospital
> domestics, the radiotherapists, the physiotherapists and so on?
> (Letter from Aneurin Bevan to Sir Walter Citrine, quoted by
> Klein 1983: 21–2)

When coupled with the desire to avoid any possible accusation of political bias in appointments, the result was a set of nominations which virtually eliminated any labour movement interests and produced a structure controlled by consultants and by former governors of the voluntary hospitals (Webster 1988: 450, 455).

A handful of nurses were appointed to these new bodies. The original boards included 13 nurses but they dwindled to 7 in 1956 and 1 in 1974. This may reflect the increasing difficulty of deflecting demands from other groups of workers for comparable representation (Webster 1988: 448). By contrast the medical profession, whose goodwill was more eagerly sought and whose opposition set a high price for co-operation, obtained 29 per cent of the appointments in 1947 and increased this to 31 per cent in 1956 (Webster 1988: 450). The risk of such a strong producer interest distorting the service to suit its own priorities led the Guillebaud Committee, which reported on the cost of the NHS in 1956, to urge a ceiling of 25 per cent on medical representation.

If nursing received scant attention at this level of administration, little is known about its influence through local management channels. There was great variation in the extent to which HMCs consulted matrons and delegated powers to their officers but further research is needed before any general patterns can be described. The ministry suggested that RHBs and HMCs should set up professional advisory groups. This practice was universally adopted for medicine, as a result of BMA pressure, and these bodies acquired considerable executive authority. They were less common and much less powerful in nursing. The RCN showed little interest and the committees which were established seldom had a majority nurse membership (White 1985: 245).

At national level, however, there was an elaborate professional advisory machinery. The 1946 Act had provided for a Central Health Services Advisory Council, which set up a number of specialist Standing Advisory Committees. Nursing was the subject of one, maternity and midwifery another and mental health, including mental nursing, a third.

The Standing Nursing Advisory Committee (SNAC) had a narrow majority of nurses – 12 out of 22 members in 1949. At this stage relatively little is known about its actual impact on ministry policy. It was certainly one of the more active committees with a regular programme of quarterly meetings. In the first ten years of its existence it dealt with a wide variety of topics from nursing techniques to cross infection, the selection of nurses and the employment of juveniles in hospitals. A number of these, such as the staffing problems of TB sanatoria and the use of enrolled nurses in mental and mental deficiency hospitals were clearly divisive issues. Some were certainly translated into ministry policy, such as the proposal for the Joint Board of Clinical Nursing

Studies which originated in a report from a SNAC sub-committee.

This last raises some important and as yet unanswerable questions about the relationship between the ministry and the GNC. The SNAC dealt with a number of educational issues and seems to have functioned as an alternative source of advice to the ministry on such matters. It is notable that the GNC failed to gain control of post-basic nursing education in this period, not only in the clinical studies courses taken over by the Joint Board in 1970 but also in the reforms of health visitor and district nurse certification during the 1960s. This suggests that the ministry may have been as concerned as in the inter-war period to prevent the strengthening of professional control over educational policy to the detriment of service needs. The proposal to second all general nursing students for TB experience, for instance, was presented to the GNC for educational approval only after it had obtained support in the SNAC as a remedy for staffing difficulties.

In addition to the advisory committees, the ministry also had a small Nursing Division, created during the war to oversee the direction of labour. This was staffed by administrative civil servants advised by a central group of 5 nursing officers on the miscellaneous staff of the chief medical officer. Their duties seem to have related mainly to hospital services, although the administrative division had a more comprehensive brief. A further 12 nursing officers with public health functions worked from the ministry's regional offices. The chief nursing officer was a relatively low status post in civil service terms, being graded as a principal and, hence, reporting to ministers only through a number of higher ranking lay administrators. Although the job had become more important by the 1960s and the number of qualified nursing officers increased, it never achieved parity with the chief medical officer and his direct access to ministers as the equal of the permanent secretary. It would not appear that the nursing officers had much weight in departmental thinking, but this is a matter which requires further investigation.

In general it seems to have been assumed that nursing policy questions would be considered along with those relating to health policy in general and that nurses would accommodate themselves to whatever arrangements were made. There is then no logical or consistent pattern to the participation of nurses in the health policy process whether at the centre or at the periphery. What is also striking is the lack of evident action by nursing organizations on policy questions, especially when contrasted with the strenuous efforts of the BMA to lobby on behalf of its constituency. It is understandable that the ministry would have been reluctant to magnify its problems by volunteering consultation to other groups but it seems to have been allowed a surprisingly easy ride along this course.

The cost of caring

The one area where the importance of nursing could not be overlooked, however, was in the NHS budget. Some commentators in the 1940s expected health care expenditures to fall once the new scheme had dealt with the accumulated backlog of disorders neglected because of the cost of treatment. Although cost questions had been raised in early cabinet discussions of the NHS, they had not been seen as a serious problem (Webster 1988: 193). Once the service came into operation, though, its financial implications horrified Labour and Conservative governments alike. Expenditures consistently outran estimates. The process was led by the hospital sector and a large share of this was contributed by the cost of nursing salaries.

In fact, a good deal of the problem reflected the failure of the treasury to adjust to inflation as a normal fact of economic life. Throughout the pre-war period prices had been stable or falling, until the impact of rearmament expenditure from 1936 onwards. While the experience of 1914–18 had led planners to expect a substantial measure of wartime inflation, it was believed that this was an abnormal condition which could be remedied by appropriate economic policies, particularly the control of wages and of public expenditure. In the event, inflation continued more or less unchecked throughout the post-war years. For this reason, the growth in maintenance expenditure shown in Table 2 actually translates into a negligible real increase in NHS resources.

The early years of the health service did see a once for all expansion in nursing establishments and a levelling up of salaries as a more uniform national approach to staffing and pay was introduced and an attempt made to remedy the pre-war depression in this industry. As it became clear that inflation was not falling generally, however, treasury orthodoxy dictated a close review of large public expenditure commitments. Within the NHS, this meant the hospital sector and, within that, the large element represented by wages and salaries. These pressures became particularly acute with the outbreak of the Korean War and the need to finance Britain's participation in the UN effort (Webster 1985: 10–11). Real wage increases for nurses, outstripping both the Retail Price Index and the Ministry of Labour Index of Wages, embarrassed a government which was seeking wage restraint in the

Table 2 Nursing salaries as a proportion of maintenance expenditure in the hospital service (England and Wales 1949–56)

	1949/50	%	1950/1	%	1951/2	%	1952/3	%	1953/4	%	1954/5	%	1955/6	%
Total maintenance expenditure	205.6		227.2		246.3		256.9		269.7		281.1		305.0	
Total wages and salaries	119.3	58.0	132.8	58.5	141.8	60.2	154.5	60.2	162.1	60.1	172.7	61.4	186.2	61.8
Breakdown of wages and salaries:														
Medical	22.0	18.4	25.6	19.3	25.0	17.6	26.0	16.8	27.2	16.0	30.8	17.8	31.7	17.0
Nursing	45.2	37.9	49.1	37.0	51.1	36.0	56.2	36.4	59.2	36.5	62.6	36.2	68.7	36.8
Other	52.1	43.7	58.1	43.7	65.7	46.4	72.2	46.8	75.8	46.7	79.3	46.0	85.7	46.2
Nursing salaries as % of total maintenance expenditure		22.0		21.6		20.7		21.9		21.9		22.3		22.5

Source: Adapted from Webster 1988: 259 (Columns may not total 100% where percentages have been rounded)

private sector and considering a freeze in the public sector (Webster 1985: 7).

In the short term, there was a debate about whether pay settlements should be included within the attempts to set ceilings on NHS expenditure, so that they would have to be met by other savings, or whether there should be automatic supplementation (Webster 1985: 9). Aneurin Bevan, the minister, also initiated the first of numerous ministerial attempts to sway the pay negotiations in the relevant Whitley Council in compliance with the government's incomes policy.

He was aided in this by the divisions on the staff side. Although there was agreement between employers and employee organizations about the importance of offering competitive salaries, there were considerable differences over the optimal package for achieving this. The trade unions pressed for improved starting salaries for students in the expectation that this would then allow them to establish a higher baseline for the whole pay structure. They also hoped that this would attract students into membership. The RCN, however, continued to exclude students from full membership and pursued its traditional objective of trying to widen differentials between trained and untrained staff. In the early years of the service, the employers favoured the position put forward by the trade unions although they had a minority of seats on the employee side of the council. As cost concerns mounted, though, the employers were able to allow the RCN to use its majority of employee seats to suppress claims with more substantial implications, either because of their absolute size or because of the number of staff involved.

As the scale of their contribution to the costs of the NHS became apparent, nursing salary budgets were an obvious target for containment. The result was a substantial long-term decline in the pay of nurses relative to that of other occupations. The pay of female nurses was 13 per cent above the average for women in the lower professional groups in 1955–6, but only 2 per cent above in 1960. Nurses' pay was 68 per cent of the national average wage in 1955–6 but only 60 per cent in 1960. The real value of a trained nurse's pay fell from £475 p.a. in 1949 to £418 p.a. in 1958 (Smail and Gray 1982). Although their wages were no longer depressed by the precarious solvency of the voluntary hospitals, nurses found themselves equally vulnerable to the chronic problems of maintaining public services in a stagnant national economy.

The Labour Government tried one sort of remedy in 1951 by introducing charges for some NHS services in the hope of discouraging demand and raising extra revenues. The Conservatives tried another in 1953, when Iain MacLeod set up a committee under Claude Guillebaud, a distinguished economist, to investigate NHS costs. Their report, in 1956, produced the politically inconvenient conclusion that there was no evidence of widespread extravagance in the NHS and, indeed, warned of further heavy expenditure in prospect to remedy the lack of post-war investment. The ministry was forced to settle for the longer haul of extracting greater efficiency from existing resources by improved management.

This task had to be accomplished against a background of growing industrial unrest. There had been stirrings in the mental hospitals during the 1950s (see pp. 138–9), but the impact of government incomes policies in the 1960s provoked a significant transformation in the formerly quiescent general hospitals. This was most striking in the RCN, whose character had begun to change with the removal of many of its restrictions on membership in 1960 and its ability to compete more effectively with the TUC-affiliated unions for recruits. The changes in 1960 had been provoked by the effects of the Nurses Act 1957 which abolished the supplementary registers and substituted a single register divided into distinct parts. By removing the basis for the RCN's restrictive policies on membership, it opened the way for the college to recruit men and to organize in the traditionally more militant areas of mental nursing. We shall discuss some of these developments in more detail later because there is a case to be argued that the changing basis of industrial relations in the NHS owed as much to contemporary fashions in management as it did to the unions or the college themselves.

Employee anger was first aroused by the freeze imposed by the Conservative Government in 1961 on pay claims by public sector workers. After a six month pause, nurses were offered a 2.5 per cent increase. This provoked widespread, although separate, campaigns by COHSE and the RCN and an appeal to the Industrial Court which awarded a flat-rate 7.5 per cent increase (Carpenter 1985: 44–6). Although the Labour Party pledged itself in opposition to an overhaul of the Whitley Council system to prevent nurses again being victims of its ponderous procedures at a time of pay restraint, this did not materialize after they were elected to office in 1964. In fact, their own pay policy created similar grievances in 1969 and pushed the RCN into its 'Raise the Roof' campaign which, as we shall show in Chapter 10 (pp. 204–5), was indirectly responsible for the creation of the Briggs Committee.

Under these twin pressures of industrial mobilization and cost containment, policy-makers turned to industrial and commercial models in the search for closer control of NHS workers. As the largest single group of employees, nurses were inevitably singled out for special attention. The Committee on Senior Nurse Staffing (Salmon), which reported in 1966 was the result (Ministry of Health 1966, cf. Carpenter 1977a: 176). It was the logical corollary of the ministry's ambitious plans for hospital building to make good the deficiencies identified by the Guillebaud Report (Ministry of Health 1966: 19). The Salmon structure was intended both to modernize nursing management to fit the new environments of the planned District General Hospitals and to achieve more efficient use of nursing labour. It was based on a division between three tiers of responsibility: top management was to participate in the determination of hospital policy; the middle tier would translate these plans into operational programmes in a particular sector, using both managerial and clinical expertise; and first line managers would have executive functions in ensuring that the work was carried out according to plan. A parallel scheme was later recommended by the Mayston Committee for local authority nursing (DHSS 1970).

Both structures were an important step towards the eventual reorganization of the service in 1974. They permitted an easy fusion of the administration of nursing in the two parts of the system that delivered most of it and anticipated much of the spirit of consensus management that we shall examine in Chapter 10 (pp. 211–12). For the first time nurses had a management system that could give them parity with other interests in the NHS. But the occupation's cool reception of these changes also indicated some of the problems ahead. Many nurses did not fit comfortably into the roles created by Salmon and Mayston and the increasing influence of professionalist ideals obstructed the development of the clinical aspects of the structure. Pembrey (1980), for instance, identified the ward sister as the key figure in the management of patient care and criticized the Salmon structure for inhibiting the development of an autonomous clinical role at this level. As Runciman (1983) points out, though, there was also a far more traditional source of opposition in the sister/consultant axis. The introduction of Salmon further compounded the conflict which we discussed earlier (pp. 56–8), when the matron's office first developed as a rival source of power in the nineteenth century hospital.

But perhaps the most significant change, although the least discussed, was the progressive dilution of nursing by the development of a range of lower-level staff to carry out many of the less technical aspects of personal care. The importance of this was highlighted by Abel-Smith (1960: 161–75, 228–39) but it has received little subsequent attention. He pointed out that the idea of formally recognizing a second-tier nurse had first been canvassed by the 1905 Select Committee on Registration but had been steadfastly opposed by nursing leaders. Only under the special conditions of the Second World War had it been possible to give official recognition to this grade. The Rushcliffe Committee established a salary scale and the Civil Nursing Reserve provided training. It became obvious that the ministry was committed to a long-term role for such personnel. In a move reminiscent of the unification of nurses against VADs in the registration debates of 1919, the RCN abandoned its outright opposition to the idea in the hope of gaining some influence over its post-war development.

In 1940, the RCN sent a deputation to the Minister of Health to press for legislative control of the assistant nurse (Abel-Smith 1960: 170). In November 1941, the college set up a Nurses Reconstruction Committee under the chairmanship of Lord Horder to consider implementation of the Athlone Committee's report. The first section of the report was devoted to the assistant nurse and declared the assistant nurse as an integral part of the profession who should become one of the most stable elements in a national nursing service (Abel-Smith 1960: 170).

The solution to competition from the assistant nurse was incorporation within the regulatory machinery of nursing. Formal recognition of the assistant nurse's status was initiated by a desire to protect the status of the registered nurse. The legitimation of a lower stratum of nursing labour would then free the student nurse to pursue an educationally orientated form of training. Thus the assistant nurse could provide the key to registered nurse professionalization. The Nurses Act 1943 provided for the GNC to create and maintain a roll of assistant nurses, absorbing existing staff and providing for a two-year training for new entrants.

The choice of the GNC as a regulatory body brought some criticism in parliament, precisely because of the fear that registered nurses might abuse their power to create such a limited and restrictive entry that the object of the reform would be defeated. This fear was not entirely without foundation: the council's initial proposals were heavily criticized as over-ambitious and the first tests were not conducted until 1949. Numbers were slow to build up and failed to match the rate of retirement of women enrolled under the *bona fide* provisions of the 1943 Act. It is possible that this contributed to the tensions in the relationship between the ministry and the GNC that are hinted at by the uses of the SNAC which we discussed earlier.

115

The result was the unplanned growth of what Abel-Smith dubbed the 'third portal', the nursing auxiliary. The Wood Committee which reviewed nursing education for the ministry in 1947 had identified a role for a grade with a much shorter and more practical training than the SEN, which might not even merit legislative recognition or regulation. As Abel-Smith points out, this was effectively the route by which what we have called the handywoman class continued to provide much of the direct care of patients, especially the chronic sick. By 1958, there were 50 per cent more of these unqualified nurses in general hospitals than there were enrolled nurses. There were more untrained staff working in the hospitals than there had been before the war. Despite the opposition of registered nursing interests, the hospitals simply could not manage without such people. After a bitter conflict on the Whitley Council, the employers officially recognized this fact in 1955 by defining the grade and attaching a pay scale to it. In the end, Abel-Smith observed, the leaders of the occupation had failed to recognize the most telling fact: for all their aspirations most direct care of the sick is provided by unqualified people for each other in their own homes. There is no particular reason why similar tasks have to be performed by a highly paid professional just because the sick person happens to be in hospital. The obstruction of more systematic training and a properly defined role for auxiliaries under the supervision of registered nurses merely denied patients such benefits as more skilful practical carers could have brought them.

The registered nurses' hostility to the use of assistants and auxiliaries has remained an important dimension of nursing politics since Abel-Smith's work was published. Despite the continued growth in the numbers of staff employed in these supporting roles during the 1960s and 1970s, the occupational leadership has remained set on eliminating them or reducing their status to that of hospital domestics. This issue will also be examined further in Chapter 10 (pp. 226–8) and its survey of the contemporary state of nursing policy.

Nursing education and the National Health Service

Before leaving this review of the impact of nationalization on general nursing, however, it is important to consider briefly the developments in nursing education which it brought about. The ministry had set up a working party, the Wood Committee, in January 1946 to review post-war provision for the recruitment and training of nurses in the context of moves towards the establishment of the NHS. Its main objectives were to deal with the nursing shortage in anticipation of increased demands from the new service and to propose ways in which the administration of nurse education could be reorganized to fit the new structure. In 1948, the committee produced its plans for an integrated system of training embracing all parts of the register. A common core lasting eighteen months would be followed by a six-month specialization in one field. Within this students would be guaranteed a forty-hour week and 'liberal' holiday periods. The reduction in length would be achieved by the elimination of repetitive work and higher educational expectations. Student placements on wards would be directed strictly towards educational objectives. The system would be organized on a regional basis, with training schools grouped into units under a director or principal rather than a hospital matron.

The nursing organizations had not been consulted by the working party during its deliberations and their reactions were predominantly hostile. The RCN (1948), in particular, objected to the reduction in training length and argued for the virtues of repetitive task performance as a method of learning. They were also unhappy about the proposal to phase out the newly acknowledged role of the assistant nurse in favour of a scheme of nursing orderlies with a three- to six-month training. Similar views were expressed in a memorandum from the GNC (1948). Both organizations similarly opposed the diminished role of hospital matrons.

> The (General Nursing) Council cannot accept the suggestion that training units should be under the control of independent Directors rather than that of the Matron of the principal hospital in each training unit. The proposed dissociation of responsibility would result in the loss of much that experience has proved of the greatest value in the training of nurses. (GNC 1948: 6)

The precise nature of this loss is nowhere more clearly specified.

It is difficult to interpret this debate without more work on the original papers. However, it is an interesting paradox that the occupational associations should be so resistant to a ministry initiative which would have concentrated the skilled elements of their work and drawn a much clearer boundary between themselves and their assistants or helpers. Indeed, the Wood proposals have a remarkably modern flavour in their model of the division of labour. The nursing organizations seem almost Luddite in their opposition to a strengthening of the educational aspects of training and its constitution as the business of a separate organization not dominated by service priorities. Some of this may be attributable to the importance of the three-year training as a symbol of professionalization. There is nothing magical about this particular time period: like any vocational training its length is dictated as much by custom and practice as by any coherent principle. More to the point may be the sort of attitudes picked out by the *Lancet* and Athlone investigations which treated nurse training as a mortifying experience during which girls were purified for their calling. The pointless repetition of mindless tasks was important as a system of discipline which could be used to identify and purge dissident elements. It was the weakening of this control which the leadership feared. We shall argue in Chapter 10 that it eventually declined only when new technologies and strategies of discipline were developed, just as National Service, a similar system of control, came to be seen as irrelevant either to the specialist skills of modern warfare or to the ordering of the nation's young men.

This view receives some support from the working party's own comments on the GNC, which may also be a useful indicator of the ministry's opinion of that body in the late 1940s and early 1950s. The Wood Report explicitly recommended using the Standing Advisory Committee for Nursing and a strengthened Nursing Division as its main sources of advice on nurse education. The GNC

> was not favourably placed to lay down and implement an educational policy for the nursing profession . . . they have very little educational representation and no counterpart to the academic representation on the GMC. (Ministry of Health 1947: 68)

The working party also criticized the dominance of matrons from large former voluntary hospitals on the council and the under-representation of municipal hospital and public health interests. The GNC and the RCN (1948: 11) reacted strongly to these charges, although the latter did concede that educational representation was inadequate. Their combined opposition was sufficient to dilute the implementation of the Wood recommendations in the Nurses Act 1949, although its analysis clearly continued to have a significant influence on ministry policy.

The Nurses Act 1949 was an essential package of legislative change, adapting the finance and administration of nurse education to the statutory framework of the NHS.[3] In this respect it has certain affinities with the Nurses Registration Act 1919 and its tidying up of nursing in the context of proposals for more general reform. The 1949 Act divided responsibility for training costs between Area Nurse Training Committees (ANTCs) in each Regional Board, administering funds channelled through the GNC for tutorial and secretarial salaries and certain equipment, and hospital budgets, which were responsible for the much larger cost of training allowances to students. Nurse membership of the GNC was restricted to those still in practice and there were minor changes to the register itself. The separate male register was amalgamated with the general register and the council was given the power to close supplementary parts. The GNC was also authorized to approve experimental training courses.

Overall, the practical impact of these changes was limited. The administration of exchequer funds for training by the GNC had the effect of strengthening ministry control, particularly evident in the struggle between the two bodies over the council's desire to introduce minimum educational requirements for entry to nursing courses, a move which was not finally accomplished until 1962. The increased recognition of male nurses was not founded on any explicit policy for reconstructing the gender composition of the occupation and had little impact until the managerial reforms of the 1960s created new opportunities for mobile and career-oriented men (Dingwall 1979).

The powers to approve experimental training courses were used cautiously. In the immediate aftermath of the war, shortened courses were offered to those who had acquired some experience of nursing with the forces or the Civil Nursing Reserve (Ministry of Health 1949–53). Later developments included shortened courses for those wanting to train for a second part of the register and for graduates. All of these were essentially simply more rapid and intensive versions of traditional courses, rather than being based on any fundamental rethinking of the nature and objectives of nursing education. A few combined university education with a nursing qualification. These tended to be slightly more innovative but remained constrained by the GNC's conservative response to the alleged problem of wastage. Much of the council's effort in the late 1950s and early 1960s was directed to identifying the 'causes' of the steady loss of recruits. However, rather than treating this as a phenomenon generated by the traditional structures of nursing and their conflict with the changing roles of women in the wider society, the council concentrated on refining methods of selection. The responsibility for wastage was pinned on individuals rather than being shared with the organization in which they worked (Dingwall 1974). In effect, the GNC left the student labour system intact and endorsed the reliance on rote learning and uncritical

119

acceptance of established authority which had formed the basis of a servant's education in Victorian or Edwardian England.

Although this service-oriented model might have been thought likely to commend itself to the ministry, it seems that the latter were more attracted to the Wood approach. The GNC line could be seen as unnecessarily costly, in that it committed the NHS to a large workforce with a modest level of education and a disproportionately long gap between entry and certification. Wood had envisaged a smaller workforce with more developed skills and a shorter training period which would allow recruits to work without supervision more quickly. They would be supplemented by semi-skilled assistants who could be trained and employed more flexibly in response to the changing patterns of demand for care. The ministry was concerned with the overall labour demand for care-providers, while the GNC was concerned with the supply of nurses. A hint of the ministry's preferences is provided by the separate provision under the Joint Board for Clinical Nursing Studies which was not placed under GNC control and which emphasized the provision of training in short, skill-specific modules throughout a nurse's career as the demands of the service changed.

It was the concern about the flexibility of care provision that the nursing organizations were slow to grasp, even when they did accept the need to separate education and service more distinctly. The Royal College of Nursing became committed to this course with its 1964 report (the Platt Report) on the reform of nurse education. Full 'student' status for nurses was seen as the magic solution to wastage and labour supply shortages. Nevertheless, the line remains a modernization of the traditionally elitist programme of the college and their desire to attract the right class of recruit, '. . . nursing must be able to offer a course which can attract and retain students who might otherwise have chosen to go to university or some other form of higher education' (RCN 1964: 12). Once again, it was an educational solution to an organizational problem. Now, however, it was linked to the need to equip the nurse to assume the responsibilities of leadership (RCN 1964: 10).

But, once again, the RCN failed to judge the mood of its audience in its commitment to the idea that training was a one-off experience in which the intake would be sifted for its higher potential and a select few cultivated for achievement. This view of vocational, or, indeed, any form of education, was already in decline by 1964 and the Platt report was further compromised by the progress towards health service reorganization. Although its exact shape and form were still undecided, few commentators were in any doubt that organizational reform was both necessary and inevitable. This would unavoidably impose changes on the nature of nursing work that could invalidate Platt-type reforms. Once again, as in 1919 and 1946, the expectation was that nursing would be reconstructed to fit a new system of health care delivery, rather than being planned with it.

It is particularly instructive to compare the approach to nursing in the 1960s with the approach to the medical profession. This was the subject of a Royal Commission set up in 1965 and reporting in 1968. The Todd Report specifically related the organization and content of medical education to the changing pattern of health care needs and the movement towards greater integration of hospital, general practitioner and local authority services. Its recommendations emphasized the interdependence of medical education and health service needs, where the Platt Report stressed the benefits for individual nurses and the international prestige of British nursing (RCN 1964: 12). The public interest was vaguely asserted, '. . . meeting the demands of the community in a highly developed country' (RCN 1964: 1). These were identified with carrying out and teaching the 'complex and exacting techniques (which) have become an established part of the treatment of patients' (RCN 1964: 10). In other words, the case for change was again derivative from and driven by changes in medical technology. But the relative balance of private over public interest left few arguments for use in persuading the ministry to take the proposals seriously.

By the mid-1960s, nursing and the NHS were in a state of some disarray. Governments had failed to get a real grip on the scale of revenue and capital investment required to provide a high-quality health care system from public revenues. Although some modest progress had been made with investment under the Hospital Plan, this had been at the expense of depressing staff wages even further. The resulting unrest was a severe embarrassment to a Labour Government committed to the reform and modernization of major British institutions by discussion and consensual change. If nursing were to play its part in this process, the workforce must be pacified and prepared for its role in a service that would be better equipped to manage its resources and to deploy new investment.

Those events will be the subject of our concluding discussion, in Chapter 10. Before exploring the contemporary history of nursing, however, we now propose to sketch the separate histories of the occupations which have fused with general nursing to create its modern form. In doing so, we hope to bring out the historic bases of some current conflicts and to offer a different perspective from the triumphalist accounts of general nursing. The struggles over fusion also help to explain some of the anxieties about specialization in the present day. Where the joint is so uncertain, it may always fracture.

Chapter seven

Mental Disorder and Mental Handicap

Adaptation of the mechanisms of social control to the needs of industrialized society affected human minds as much as human bodies. Chapter 2 discussed the developments in medical knowledge which produced more standardized conceptions of what body states would count as health and illness and the search for ways of enforcing those new definitions throughout the society. Modern conceptions of mental disorder and mental handicap were produced out of the same process. A new form of society called for a reconstruction of the way people thought about their relationships to nature and to each other.

Mental disorder had to be thought into existence as a way of describing certain sorts of behaviour and the states of mind that could be inferred from them. Under the particular influence of the writing of Michel Foucault (1965), Whig accounts of medical progress gave way to a critical examination of the ways in which people had written about the human mind and the assumptions which were embedded into those accounts. It was argued that the industrial and political revolutions of the late eighteenth and early nineteenth centuries had led to a thoroughgoing redefinition of what constituted orderly behaviour. The reconstruction outlined in Chapter 2 was as much mental as it was moral. But, by treating the causes of disorder as defects of biology rather than as intentional or wilful, the implied rejection of the new ways of ordering perception and behaviour lost any legitimacy. It could be seen as a quirk of nature over which the individual had no control rather than as a deliberate challenge to the social order. Thus, according to Foucault the problem was assigned to the medical profession rather than to the justice system.

The contests over the interpretation of the history of mental disorder have largely been fought around the issues of psychiatric knowledge and of the rise of psychiatry as a medical specialty. The history of nursing care for the mentally sick and the mentally handicapped, 'lunatics' and the 'feeble-minded' to use an older vocabulary, has remained substantially untouched by this revisionism. Yet it probably has far more to say about the experience of patients than any study of medical sources. In the old asylums with their handful of medical staff under a remote superintendent, the attendants would have had a critical role as intermediaries between the theories of the day and the ordinary life of the institution.

Asylums

Before the 1830s, the mentally disordered were dealt with in a relatively informal manner (Macdonald 1981, Porter 1983). Although mental capacity had been a matter of interest to lawyers for generations (Unsworth 1987: 36–58), because of its importance to questions about the management of property or the intention underlying alleged crimes, it had mostly been defined in practice by the inability to fulfil available roles in the local community. The response depended a great deal on the resources available to the victim's family and the nature of the threat which the disordered behaviour represented to others. In a well-off household, a disordered family member might simply be dealt with by extra attention from the domestic servants. Paupers might receive outdoor relief or another villager might be paid to care for them. Only a small minority were confined to institutions.

The situation changed radically with the Poor Law Amendment Act, 1834, which paved the way for a greatly enlarged national system of workhouses. As Chapter 2 described, these institutions initially absorbed all types of destitute paupers. But the increasingly prevalent theory that many types of mental deficiency and insanity could be cured by the correct medical treatment led fairly quickly to the development of a separate system of asylums.

Although the asylums were distinct from the workhouses, both reflected the unified model of organizational provision evolved by the Victorians to deal with paupers, delinquents and other economically unproductive groups (Busfield 1986, Doerner 1981, Mellett 1982, Scull 1979, 1981). Workhouses, prisons, and asylums were physically similar and served overlapping functions. The same case might end up in any of them, depending upon the vagaries of local admission and transfer policies, the definitions and explanations of rule-breaking behaviour currently in fashion. The whole institutional system was designed to provide minimum standards of care consistent with the principles of control, economy, and less eligibility discussed in Chapter 2. The struggles to increase medical influence in the general workhouses have already been mentioned, but the early ascription of a biological origin to mental disorder established a bias towards medical control in the asylums from an early date. The medical profession's claim to offer scientific criteria for the classification and treatment of cases, according to the same logic that they were introducing to the study of physical illnesses, was a clinical extension of the principles of rational economic management which dominated the rest of the system.

At first there was little discrimination between the feeble-minded and the insane, but the development of distinct voluntary sector provisions for each was gradually reflected in the public facilities. By the end of the century, the specialists in psychological medicine controlled an elaborate taxonomy of rule-breaking or deviant behaviour. This expertise was a considerable source of power in a society which had become haunted by fears of racial degeneration.[1] Whatever the justification for these concerns, they made relevant expert knowledge a basis for considerable professional authority (cf. Freidson 1986). Although the medical superintendents were not as rich as the most successful consultant physicians, their administrative and medical power was spectacular. A medical superintendent was the unchallenged master of the entire institution, often a rather remote country estate which might extend to 600 acres with its own farm and workshops both contributing to its self-sufficiency and compounding its isolation.

The numbers involved were substantial. In 1859, the county asylums held 16,000 patients. By 1939, the public authorities were providing places for 132,000 lunacy patients and 32,500 mental defectives. In 1930, general workhouses were still maintaining about 16,000 lunatics and 6,000 mental defectives, together with a large but indeterminable number of elderly patients suffering various mental problems associated with ageing. It can be estimated that at least 200,000 patients in public institutions were receiving mental care by 1939 (Board of Control 1915–38). This made up half of the hospital beds taken over in 1948 by the National Health Service.

Given the isolation of the institutions and the absolute power of their medical superintendents, the regime actually experienced by patients varied a great deal depending on the character and beliefs of the individual doctor in charge. It might vary from benevolent paternalism to insensitive authoritarianism. The official ethos of the British asylum movement was derived from the experiment of the Quaker community at The Retreat in York (Digby 1985). Its founder, William Tuke, had introduced the system of 'moral treatment' to this small private asylum. It was based on the theory that madness arose from an inflammation of human passions, the animal side of a person's nature (Fears, 1977, 1978). The regime stressed self-discipline and work, providing a structured and routinized environment from which any stimulus to the passions had been removed. In such an ordered world patients might find it easier to regain control of their disordered minds.

The county asylums were built to reduce the need for physical restraint, which Tuke used only for specific therapeutic purposes, and to implement this new theory of moral discipline. In practice, they were less liberal in their regimes than The Retreat. With its middle-class patients, moral treatment seems to have consisted largely of walks in the garden and reading improving books. Poorer patients were expected to help with manual labour appropriate to their station in life. Since the asylums were full of pauper patients, their regimes depended from the start much more on exacting obedience than encouraging self-control and self-rehabilitation. Tuke's notions about the therapeutic value of work were used to justify the forced labour of asylum industries intended to minimize the burden on the Poor Rate. Like workhouses, asylums were the reverse side of the drive against outdoor relief.

Despite the humanitarian language, then, control in the county asylums involved intense disciplinary pressure on patients, reinforced by punishment, segregation and physical or chemical restraint. By the 1870s, for instance, there was considerable concern about the way in which new sedatives were being used in place of positive moral treatment (Busfield 1986: 261, 263, Digby 1985: 122–30, Russell 1984: 95–8, Santos and Stainbrook 1949: 70–1). Whether benign or harsh, however, the actual execution of the medical superintendent's policies was largely in the hands of his staff of attendants.

Asylum attendants

Initially, asylum staff were indiscriminately called 'keepers', 'superintendents', or 'attendants'. The last of these eventually became the preferred term for male staff, while 'nurse' was a title reserved for women. From the outset asylum work was dominated by working-class men, the nearest equivalent of the 'handywoman' class in general nursing. This resulted partly from the need for physical strength if patients needed to be forcibly restrained. However, the importance of the economic activities of the asylum should not be overlooked. These men had the kind of low-level skills of agriculture and related workshop production which were essential for the supervision of patient labour. The declining demand for workers in the agricultural sector which freed women for employment in general nursing also released men for the staffing of asylums.

Wages and conditions were modelled on those of domestic or farm servants. At the end of the nineteenth century an attendant might typically be paid about £30 per annum while a medical superintendent could be earning £1,000 (Digby 1985: 142–4, Hunter and Macalpine 1974: 93, Russell 1984: 305–19, Walton 1981: 180–1 cites more generous attendant scales at Lancaster). Attendants worked long days, slept in on a rota basis and received little time off. Night staff were gradually introduced from about 1860 (Hunter and Macalpine 1974: 96–7). But 14-hour days, 84-hour weeks and as little as one day off a month were still commonplace in 1900 (Board of Control 1925: 40–3).

This social isolation was compounded by the strict disciplinary control exerted over staff. Even at The Retreat, attendants were subject to the discipline typical of any large domestic establishment (Digby 1985: 140–70). In the pauper asylums the attendants shared the conditions of the patients. Both were equally subject to the same complex web of rules and to the expectation of automatic and unquestioning obedience. Although the theory of moral treatment might have envisaged a creative role for attendants, the staffing levels would always have made this difficult to implement. Most asylums varied between staffing ratios of 1:15, and 1:25, depending on the nature of the patients. Since the conditions were unattractive, asylums rarely succeeded in their aspirations to recruit intelligent, kind, industrious and creative attendants. The priority afforded to internal control tended to mean they engaged ignorant and heavy-handed disciplinarians who were unemployable elsewhere and could only be kept in check by a regime that further diminished whatever possibility there might have been for attendant initiative.

There were periodic complaints from medical superintendents about the quality of the staff available to them but few sustained attempts to improve the situation until the 1890s. As with general nursing, it was a shift in medical practice that created the conditions for occupational development. The early enthusiasm for treatment of the mentally disordered had dissipated in the face of its limited success. Feeble-mindedness, in particular, was recognized as irreversible by medical means, although efforts continued to be directed to the training of the mentally handicapped so that the burden of care might be reduced (Pritchard 1963: 54–62). Moral treatment, in practice, amounted to little more than containment. However, towards the end of the century, doctors turned again to the search for an organic basis to mental disorder in the hope of finding more effective remedies. Moral therapy gave way to physical treatments such as baths, showers, wet packing, medical electricity, and the administration of drugs. This reframing of mental disorder as a disease of the mind exactly analogous to diseases of the body generated a demand for assistants with a better grasp of underlying biological principles so that they could give more effective aid to the doctors.

In order to achieve this, the medical superintendents began to introduce the model of general hospital nursing into the asylums. At The Retreat, for example, nursing uniforms were introduced during the 1890s, along with a nursing hierarchy modelled on general hospital structures. Attempts were made to require some formal education of the staff (Digby 1985: 168). Some asylums tried to recruit general-trained nurses. Matron posts in asylums offered one way for ambitious women to circumvent the promotion blockages created by the appointment of relatively young candidates to senior posts in the general sector. The most important development, however, was the introduction of an examination for a national certificate in 1891 by the Medico-Psychological Association, a professional organization dominated by medical superintendents.

Experiments with the training of attendants had been carried out by individual superintendents since 1845 (Walk 1961). In 1885 a group of Scottish superintendents produced a 64-page text, *Handbook for the Instruction of Attendants on the Insane*. This was adopted in a revised and expanded form by the MPA in 1893. Significantly, most of the enlargement consisted of additional material relating to general anatomy, physiology and nursing. With the addition of self-assessment questions and information about training and examinations in 1896, this volume became the required text for the MPA certificate course. It continued to be revised through seven editions until 1923, when the title was changed to *Handbook for Mental Nurses*, reflecting the general acceptance of this new designation for staff of both sexes. This edition remained the standard work on the subject until 1954. Because red covers were used from 1885 onwards, this text was known as the 'Red Handbook' and it assumed canonical importance in mental nursing education for the best part of a century. A register of successful candidates in the examination was maintained by the MPA. The MPA certificate became an attractive qualification. In 1891 there were 35 successful candidates in the examination and this increased rapidly to an annual average of around 600. By 1924, 17,429 certificates had been issued, although only 26 per cent of male staff and 16 per cent of female staff employed in that year possessed the qualification (Board of Control 1924: 10). In 1934, only 30 per cent of all staff in mental deficiency institutions held the certificate. The support of the medical superintendents ensured that the MPA certificate was preferred over the rival GNC qualification until the 1950s as a route to career advancement.

Attendants thus became the first segment of nursing to acquire a relatively uniform system of training and examination and a register of certified practitioners, although these were imposed on them rather than achieved by their own lobbying initiatives. The initial impetus towards occupational organization also came from the medical superintendents with their sponsorship of the foundation of an Association of Workers in Asylums (AWA) in 1897. But these developments had only a limited impact on the nature and status of the care of the mentally disordered. The pay was insufficient to attract skilled and career-oriented men. To the extent that such recruits came forward, they tended to be men who had retired from pensionable occupations such as the police or the armed forces, and who were not wholly dependent on their income from nursing. The conditions of service, especially the social isolation and low regard for the patients, prevented mental nursing from sharing in the small pool of more educated women who were drawn into the general hospitals. To the extent that such women were brought into senior posts, they incurred the resentment of attendants who saw their own prospects being blocked. Developments in education, training and professional organization were cheaper than remedying the basic social and economic problems of staff in this sector, but they could not substitute for such measures.

Unionization

Asylum work is important, then, as much for its contribution to the unionization of nursing as to the professionalist model of occupational development. Although nurses in Poor Law infirmaries had begun to unionize from 1885, the asylums saw the most substantial growth of an industrial model of organization and were a crucial arena for the struggle between these rival modes of work orientation.

The main stimulus to unionization was the Asylum Officers Superannuation Act 1909. This Act, which was supported by the

AWA, was intended to improve the attendants' conditions of service by requiring employers to introduce pension schemes. These, however, were put on a contributory basis, although many attendants had previously enjoyed non-contributory arrangements. The result was an effective wage cut. It crystallized many of the attendants' dissatisfactions with their position relative to general nurses in the public sector who had gained non-contributory pensions, a 70-hour week and higher wages. In 1910 the male attendants formed a new National Asylum Workers Union (NAWU), leaving the AWA as mainly the representative of career-oriented female nurses (Adams 1969). The NAWU affiliated to the Labour Party in 1914 and to the TUC in 1923. By 1920, it had 15,000 members, still a minority of the workforce but making it easily the largest single representative organization for asylum staff (Carpenter 1980, 1985).

The NAWU achieved some significant gains for its members. Its original objectives were a weekly wage of £3.15s, equal pay for men and women, a 48-hour working week, state registration and joint wage bargaining (Carpenter 1980: 143). The spread of unionization led to investigations of working conditions by a House of Commons Select Committee in 1911 and by the Board of Control in 1922.[2] Unionization also stimulated the majority of Asylum Visiting Committees to combine into the Mental Hospitals Association in 1918. This was the first national organiz-ation of asylum managers as distinct from medical superintendents. As such, it was important not only for the co-ordination of collective bargaining in a new Joint Conciliation Committee but also for the sharing of management experience and the articulation of an alternative perspective on the development of the sector. Apart from its recognition as the sole employees' representative in the Joint Committee, the NAWU also obtained negotiating rights with the London County Council, which controlled the capital's asylums under separate arrangements. As a result of these developments the union succeeded in gaining a shorter working week and enhanced overtime payments although it failed to increase general wage rates, reduce urban/rural differentials or achieve equal pay (Carpenter 1985: 23–6, Ministry of Health 1945: 35–42). Unionization was relevant to the debate over registration which will be reviewed below.

Mental hospitals

The philosophy of social reconstruction after the First World War also embraced the modernization of what were now called the 'mental hospital services' (Nolan 1986: 17–18). The actual impact of reconstruction was limited by the post-war economic stagnation, which made it impossible either to replace or improve the old county asylums. Their beds were under increasing pressure from an ageing long-stay patient population. The problem was aggravated by the innovation of the Mental Treatment Act 1930 which separated the mental hospitals from the Poor Law and made it possible for patients of all classes to obtain admission on a voluntary basis. This encouraged some interest in the development of prevention, early diagnosis and aftercare through out-patient services (Board of Control 1922, 1930). But the only area where there was any substantial growth in provision was mental deficiency, following the Mental Deficiency Act 1913. This had established the separation of mental handicap and mental illness facilities as a national priority. Initial plans had called for 100,000 places to be provided, although less than half of these had been created by 1939.

The war had given a renewed impetus to the search for physical causes of mental disorder. There had been one genuine research advance in the discovery that general paralysis of the insane was the result of syphilis. If this were the case, the other disorders might be pinned down to a single organic base. This theory was also encouraged by the experience of dealing with shell-shock victims. If mental illness could affect normal, respectable individuals without prior warning, then it might be appropriate to consider it on the model of an acute medical or surgical problem. Many physical treatments were devised or rediscovered in the search for effective organic therapy. The Board of Control *Annual Report* for 1924 (pp. 13–15) lists the remedies then in fashion: verandas, continuous baths and hydrotherapy, electrical treatment, surgery, dental treatment, and X-ray treatment. There was a vogue for using deliberate infection with malaria to treat general paralysis. Between 1936 and 1939 Board of Control reports gave provisional encouragement to insulin treatment and drug induced convulsive therapy (see also Busfield 1986: 333–6).

These various developments had repercussions for the work of asylum attendants. They appeared as further justifications for the view that the care of the mentally disordered was a specialized branch of general nursing. Textbooks began to emphasize general nursing techniques, which were required by, for example, malaria or insulin therapy. Management was reshaped on the model of general hospitals and double qualification was urged on all those who aspired to senior posts.

The creation of mental nursing

The logic of the above developments might seem to point to the full assimilation of mental to general nursing, as separate branches of a common occupation. This, indeed, was embodied in the provisions of the Nurses Registration Act 1919 for the creation of a supplementary register of mental nurses. In fact, the inter-war period was marked by a more or less constant battle between the GNC and the MPA for control of the certification of nurses, a struggle which the GNC conspicuously lost.

Both the MPA and the NAWU had long wanted state registration. The MPA certificate was accepted by the GNC in 1920 for the purposes of admission to the supplementary register. But the association was reluctant to give up its own role in certification. It had been hoped that the MPA certificate would provide a foundation for a state registration examination and that there would be no serious break in the system of training (*Nursing Times*, 7 May 1921: 504). Indeed, the MPA expected to gain delegated powers to continue examining under the new legislation. When the GNC rejected this idea, the MPA decided to continue with its own certificate. The combination of medical and union support established its dominance throughout the period. The GNC examination never attracted more than 40–60 entrants at any time between the wars (Bendall and Raybould 1969: 97).

The GNC and MPA (RMPA from 1925) kept up a bitter conflict through the pages of various journals and committees of inquiry during the 1920s and 1930s. The GNC argued the case for a unified occupation and the desirability of setting a common standard for all nurses. The RMPA was blamed for all deficiencies in mental nursing (Board of Control 1925: 10–37, *Lancet Commission* 1932: 11–13, 153–5, Ministry of Health 1945: 6–7, 17–26). Mental nurses were dismissed as 'spoilt children of the MPA' (Board of Control 1922: 71–3). The RMPA claimed that its examinations had a proven value and were designed to meet the specific practical needs of mental nurses. They shared the prestige of the medical profession. The GNC, on the other hand, had only two mental nurses among its membership and could not be relied upon to be sufficiently sensitive to the special needs of this form of work. Its decision to put mental nurses on a supplementary register was interpreted as an imputation of inferiority. The RMPA capitalized on its established position as a certifying body by undercutting the GNC's examination fees. It was argued and has recently been confirmed that the RMPA course was more limited and examinations easier than those of the GNC (Nolan 1986: 21). By these means the RMPA maintained a major role in this area until 1951.

The NAWU supported the RMPA line in defence of its members' job security. It was feared that the intervention of the GNC would precipitate a flood of cheap female labour from the general hospitals into the mental institutions. The union was already under considerable pressure, like most others, from the depressed economic climate of the inter-war years. As other sources of employment dried up there occurred a short-term improvement in the quality and quantity of staff available. Staffing ratios reached the recommended level of 1:10 on both the male and the female sides of the hospitals in 1924 (Board of Control 1924: 8–10). But the mental hospitals were not insulated from the general retrenchment in public expenditure and these staffing ratios had deteriorated to 1:11 on the male side, and 1:11.8 on the female side by 1939 (Ministry of Health 1945: 47–8).

These financial problems bore heavily on pay and conditions of work in these institutions. Some improvements did occur. Many hospitals constructed separate nurses' homes for staff, although 40 per cent of nurses were still accommodated in hospital buildings in 1938 (Board of Control 1938: 13–14, Nolan 1986: 20). Working hours were reduced from 66 to 60 and later to 48 per week, although this last was strongly resisted by medical superintendents in the more remote areas, ostensibly in the interests of the continuity of care, but more probably because of its implications for staff recruitment and costs (*Lancet Commission* 1932: 158–9, Board of Control 1924: 23–40, 1925: 40–8, Ministry of Health 1945: 41–2).

Wages suffered most during this period. The joint conciliation machinery produced a complex and chaotic pay structure. The first major review, far from accepting the NAWU claim for a substantial increase, concluded that the major problem was the lack of differentials in the newly-installed nursing hierarchy. Its remedy was to cut the wages of probationers by 50 per cent and of staff nurses by a lesser amount. Equal pay was resisted, although it was accepted that the male lead should be reduced from 30 to 20 per cent. At this time, female staff nurses could be paid as little as £36 per annum whereas the national average minimum was about £60 and the maximum £80. For comparison women workers in the cotton industry rarely earned less than £100 per annum at this date (Board of Control 1924: 29–33, Ministry of Health 1945: 35–42).

Despite the early unionization of mental nurses, their economic position gradually declined relative to general nursing. The effects were most keenly felt among women nurses. In 1938, there was an overall shortage of women staff of 6 per cent, but in some areas this reached as high as 16 per cent. There were complaints about the levels of wastage and the high rates of turnover, which were attributed to unqualified female 'drifters' whose influence was alleged to discourage girls 'of a good type' from taking up the work (*Lancet Commission* 1924: 155–6, Ministry of Health 1945: 14).

But it is important not to take such complaints at face value. They may be just as much assertions of occupational ideals as of fact. Many employments which recruit large numbers of working-class women have adapted to high levels of wastage and turnover. Indeed, it may even be this flexibility of employment that attracts staff in the first place. Complaints, then, may be part of the claim to professional status, the idea that nursing is a type of work which involves a special kind of commitment rather than being judged alongside other types of skilled manual work for women. Certainly the employers did not respond by seeking more aggressively to recruit educated women by improving pay, conditions or career opportunities. Instead they turned attention to regions of high unemployment and especially to Ireland as sources of cheap labour which might be retained by insulating it from the local labour market (Ministry of Health 1945: 6–7, Nolan 1986: 20).

Histories of psychiatry derived from medical or administrative sources tend to depict the period as one of the professional maturation of the specialty. The Mental Treatment Act 1930 was variously hailed as a 'revolutionary development' or a 'great landmark' (Board of Control 1929:1, 1930). This consolidated the separation between mental hospitals and the Poor Law, and it introduced an emphasis on voluntary and preventive intervention under medical direction. It rejected the legalism of nineteenth century approaches to mental disorder in favour of psychiatric discretion. The power and prestige of psychiatry were reflected in the standing of the RMPA and the Mental Hospitals Association, as well as major voluntary organizations such as the Central Association for Mental Welfare and the Eugenics Society. The latter had a particular impact through its campaigns for the sterilization of the 'unfit'.

This interpretation of the 1930 Act has recently been questioned by Unsworth (1987), who argues that it is better interpreted as left-over business from post-war reconstruction, rather than as a radical new initiative. This impression of stagnation is also borne out by interviews with former mental nurses from this period:

> despite the efforts of some Medical Superintendents to improve the care of mental patients through the training of mental

nurses, care did not noticeably improve. Although psychiatry was generating a compassionate and scientific rhetoric, the rhetoric was limited by those who were expected to implement it. The vast majority of nursing staff were poorly educated working class people who happily settled for institutionalised life which relieved them of taking decisions or of thinking for themselves. (Nolan 1986: 21)

Not for the first time in this history, it would appear that there was a substantial gap between the Whig accounts of progress and enlightenment and the mundane reality of life on the average ward in the average mental and mental deficiency hospital. Elimination of the old nomenclature, such as 'asylum', 'lunatic' and 'idiot' should not be taken at face value. It carried no necessary connotation of progress towards a more humanitarian conception of mental disorder or handicap. Mental nursing continued much as it ever had, as a humble occupation caring for a rather heterogeneous group of people who were unable to care for themselves in the outside world.

The National Health Service

The mental health services were initially left largely unaffected by the introduction of the National Health Service. The administrative integration of this sector with other branches of public health care was merely the logical outcome of policies pursued by the Ministry of Health since 1919. In practice, the interest of Regional Hospital Boards lay elsewhere and the mental hospitals and mental deficiency institutions were starved of investment and administrative or professional initiative. The mental health services continued to moulder away in their antiquated buildings (Webster 1988: 325–40). Psychiatric medicine and mental nursing shared in this social and economic decline relative to acute medicine.

Two events are conventionally seen as critical to change in this sector. The Mental Health Act 1959 completed the dismantling of the legalism of the Lunacy Act 1890 and marked the high water mark of medical dominance in the definition and treatment of mental disorders (Jones 1960). Indeed, its dismantling of legal protections was so comprehensive that it rapidly came under counter-attack for the inadequate protection afforded to patients who had been compulsorily detained. After a long campaign by civil libertarians, a tighter framework of legal regulation was reintroduced by the Mental Health Act 1983 (Unsworth 1987).

The decade between 1955 and 1965 also saw the transformation of physical treatment by the introduction of the major tranquillizers such as chlorpromazine and reserpine, followed by anti-depressants and other psychotropic drugs. Patients could be more easily restrained by these new chemical means and the internal order of the institutions could become more relaxed (DHSS 1975: 11–12). It became realistic to think in terms of short-stay admissions as a way of containing acute episodes in continuing disorders rather than needing to keep patients in a kind of preventive detention. One indicator of the change is the way the 1964 edition of the *Handbook for Mental Nurses* devoted 16 pages to drug therapy out of the 21 allotted to the discussion of physical treatment, while the 1954 edition had only devoted 10 pages out of 45 to this aspect of the topic.

The mid 1950s marked a historic turning point in the mental health services. For the first time since the asylum system was established there commenced a downward trend in the population of the mental hospitals. The reasons for this downturn are complex. Conventionally innovations in drug treatment mentioned above are invoked as the primary factor in the situation. Drug treatment should be seen in the context of a general change in attitudes. The development of the consultant service under the NHS brought with it new therapeutic fashions and a more active approach to patient review.

The downturn in in-patient numbers was of great policy significance because it occurred precisely at a time when the government was giving its first serious thought to co-ordinating the NHS hospital planning and looking for economies to compensate for the cost of remedying the lack of capital investment in health care.

In 1962, it was decided to reduce the number of beds provided in mental hospitals from 160,000 to 80,000 within 16 years. Few believed that this was an attainable target but it was actually achieved. A few bold spirits revived the hopes of 1920 that the old asylums would be completely closed down and patients treated either in general hospitals or in the community (e.g. J. Enoch Powell in NAMH 1961: 5–10).[2] This policy of institutional contraction might have been applied with as much, if not more, justification to the care of the mentally handicapped but the inertia in that area was even greater (Ryan with Thomas 1980, Alaszewski 1983: 227–8). Its consequences for mental nursing were depressing.

Mental nursing and the NHS

Mental nursing entered the NHS in a state of crisis with low staffing levels, low morale and low wages. The increased rate of admissions in the early years of the health service placed it under further stress. A review undertaken in 1949 by the distinguished psychiatrist Aubrey Lewis, revealed a 'desperately serious' situation calling for a 'revolutionary' solution (Webster 1988: 334). A further investigation undertaken in 1954 reported that there had been no noticeable improvement. By the accepted standards – a nurse/patient ratio of 1:4.5 in mental hospitals, and 1:6 in mental deficiency hospitals – there was a shortfall of about 20 per cent in the staffing of mental deficiency hospitals and on the male side of mental hospitals, and of 35 per cent on the female side of mental hospitals. Although almost 80 per cent of male nurses were now qualified, the proportion of qualified female nurses had declined from 40 to 36 per cent between 1949 and 1953. Recruitment of student nurses was falling and the rate of wastage was rising (Webster 1988: 334). As in general nursing (see Chapter 6), the ministry tried to respond by a combination of educational reform and planned dilution through the greater use of nursing assistants.

In 1951, the RMPA, which was soon to be translated into the Royal College of Psychiatrists, was persuaded to relinquish its examining role in favour of the GNC. The exact thinking behind this decision remains obscure, but it is noticeable that the GNC simultaneously reformed its RMN syllabus to reduce its general nursing content and increase the material specifically relevant to psychiatry and psychology. These changes were taken further in the Experimental Syllabus of 1957, which was adopted as standard in 1965. This abandoned the common preliminary examination and replaced it with one specific to mental nurses (Budge 1967). The joint Mental Health and Nursing SAC report (1968), *Psychiatric Nursing Today and Tomorrow*, questioned the value of routinely seconding mental nurses for general training. Such developments invite the conclusion that some understanding had been reached about the undesirability of forcing mental nursing too firmly into the model of general nursing. The price of GNC control was its toleration of a greater degree of diversity in the occupation it regulated.

The proposal for greater use of auxiliaries had originally been put forward in the Reports of the 1924 Departmental Committee and the 1926 Royal Commission, but it had been rejected by the authors of the 1945 Report on Mental Nursing. The idea was now revived by a Ministry of Labour Advisory Committee and adopted by the Nursing and Midwifery Standing Advisory Committee of the Ministry of Health. This group, which was dominated by general hospital interests, recommended the creation of an

Enrolled Nurse grade in the mental hospitals. The suggestion met with vigorous resistance from the Mental Health Standing Advisory Committee, which represented psychiatrists. In effect, it was a continuation of the struggles of the inter-war period with the psychiatrists and the major union, now the Confederation of Health Service Employees, seeking to maintain mental nursing as a specialist area of work, while the general nurses, now with the support of the more powerful lay administrators, tried to assimilate it to the model of training and work organization thought appropriate in their sector. The generalists eventually won, as they had in the contest between the RMPA and the GNC for primacy in the certification of mental nurses. Nevertheless, the opposition was sufficiently powerful to delay the introduction of enrolled mental nurses until 1965 (Webster 1988: 335–6).

The Mental Health SAC had urged that qualified nurses and students training for the RMN should constitute at least 80 per cent of the direct patient care staff of the mental hospitals. By 1972, enrolled nurses and nursing assistants made up about 45 per cent of the nursing workforce (HMSO 1972: Table 33). The 1971 White Paper, *Better Services for the Mentally Ill*, set a target of 60 per cent for qualified psychiatric nurses, which remains an official, although as yet unrealized, goal.

The rival models for the organization of mental nursing work were reflected in different approaches to questions of pay and conditions. As in the pre-war years, the ministry preferred dilution or cosmetic devices like recruitment drives or redecorating hospital interiors to substantial expenditure on real improvements in wages or the work environment. This undoubtedly contributed to frustration of nursing staff and thereby to the growth of unionization in the mental hospitals. COHSE, the descendant of the NAWU, was formed in 1946 with 40,000 members. By 1980, it had 215,000. Carpenter (1977a, 1978) and Manson (1977) suggest that this was partly a reflection of management encouragement of union organization in the public sector in order to create a partner for the corporatist forms of industrial relations that were then fashionable.

Nevertheless, COHSE also built up a reputation as an aggressive defender of its members' interests. It caused serious embarrassment to the ministry with its picketing of the 1955 Mental Health Exhibition, which was intended to tour the country as a major showpiece for the NHS. Sporadic outbreaks of industrial action between 1955 and 1959 by its members against the frustrations of the cumbersome Whitley Council negotiating machinery paved the way for the more disruptive tactics of the next decade. These protests were the first public warning of the demoralizing conditions being experienced by staff and patients in the nation's mental hospitals (Carpenter 1985: 41–2, Webster 1988: 336–7).

The achievements of COHSE were limited and mostly gained on the tails of mobilization by general nurses. There was little progress on the issue of pay until the Halsbury Award of 1974 (Carpenter 1982: 74–90, 1985: 36–62). As in the earlier period, there was more success in gaining reductions in hours, with the working week being reduced from 42 to 40, and finally 37 hours. Without a corresponding increase in staff, the main result was a further increase in the load on those who remained.

To the degree that economic factors underlay the problems of mental nursing, the NHS failed to reverse the continuing decline in this sector. It is certainly arguable that the average mental nurse was worse off in 1980 than in 1920. The rundown of mental hospitals envisaged by the policymakers of the early 1960s had destroyed any incentive to invest in improving the dilapidated condition of old institutions, or to replace them with modern facilities. Mental nurses were effectively being told that there was no real future for their specialty. Their work was likely to become ever more burdensome as younger and less damaged patients were discharged and the hospital population whittled down to the old and the severely disordered. In consequence, the problems of poor recruitment, high wastage and staff shortages which had bedeviled these institutions since the 1920s, and before, continued unabated. Conditions in the hospitals spiralled downward, taking the nursing staff with them.

Hospitals in trouble

In these circumstances, it is hardly surprising that patient care deteriorated to a level that created the conditions for ill-treatment to occur. Such allegations form a recurrent theme in the history of lunacy (Walton 1981: 186–8). The prevention of inhumane treatment had been a concern of both the Lunacy Commissioners and the Board of Control, although the asylums were periodically shaken by allegations such as those made by Montagu Lomax in *The Experiences of an Asylum Doctor* (1921). These events invariably provoked a prompt public investigation, which usually exonerated the institution involved.

The emergence of new allegations of ill-treatment in the 1960s was particularly ironic because of the assumption that such things had been eliminated by the NHS and the enlightened regimes made possible by the Mental Health Act (1959). But correspondence in *The Times* in November 1965 signalled concern about conditions in these hospitals and this was fuelled by the specific charges made in Barbara Robb's book, *Sans Everything*, in 1967. An initial investigation dismissed these criticisms, but it was soon undercut by the findings of inquiries into particular hospitals, from the Ely Hospital Report of 1969 onwards. It emerged that institutional regimes had changed far less than fashionable psychiatric writing might imply. Custodial habits had persisted from the days of the county asylums well into the twentieth century. They represented the practical responses to the long-term deprivation of the staff in this sector. Change was blocked by insensitive bureaucracy and a rigidly hierarchical division of labour between the caring occupations, problems which were not improved by the 1974 NHS reorganization (Martin 1984, Beardshaw 1982).

The NHS was slow to respond to these problems and to make a full-hearted commitment to the new administrative practice required by changing therapeutic ideals. *Better Services for the Mentally Ill* (DHSS 1975) gave a rather belated assurance that mental hospitals would not precipitately be run down in the switch to a community-based service. But, although conceding that this transition would take a further twenty-five years to achieve, it had little positive to say about what was to happen in the meantime to hospital services. It devoted only 1 page out of 90 to mental nursing and most of this was addressed to community services. The curriculum shifts in mental nursing during the 1960s had certainly prepared the ground for transition to community care, with a greater emphasis on psychological and psychosocial aspects of mental disorder and treatment. On the other hand, notwithstanding the rapid contraction of mental hospitals, there were less than 1,000 community psychiatric nurses in 1977 and only about 2,000 in 1980, compared with some 50,000 working in hospitals (DHSS 1980: 49–50). During the same period, the number of community nurses in mental handicap increased from 50 to 300 (DHSS *Third Report* 1979–81: 23). This example simultaneously illustrates the difficulty of shifting human resources to community care and the general neglect of policy regarding the mental hospital sector.

As in earlier decades, neglect was even more conspicuous in the case of mental handicap. Circular MH 65/104, which had been produced in connection with the 1962 Hospital Plan, expressed various pious hopes about ameliorating conditions for the mentally handicapped, but went little further. *Better Services for the Mentally Handicapped* (DHSS 1971) was, then, the first major review of policy for this client group since 1929 (Ryan with

Thomas 1980: 117–8, Alaszewski 1983: 229). This document criticized the custodial tradition but a firm leadership towards community provision emerged only with the formation of the National Development Group for the Mental Handicapped (1974–9) and the Development Team for the Mental Handicapped (1976), which acted as interprofessional ginger groups within the DHSS, as well as disseminating models of practice through health authorities. The reports from these groups hint at the depth of the rift between nurses trained in very different traditions (e.g. DHSS *First Report* 1976–7: 32). The interdisciplinary thrust of policy was reflected in reports like those of the Court Committee on Child Health Services (HMSO 1976) and the Warnock Committee of Inquiry into the Education of Handicapped Children and Young People (HMSO 1978).

The weakening of occupational boundaries and the shift to community care created a serious identity crisis for nurses in the mental health services, especially in the area of mental handicap. At the outset, the first chairman of the GNC had objected to the inclusion of nurses caring for mental defectives in the registration machinery because 'they have no claim to be called Sick Nurses at all' (Sir W. P. Herringham to Sir Arthur Robinson, PRO, MH 55/463). Now the issue was revived with the Briggs Committee's recommendation that 'a new caring profession for the mentally handicapped should emerge gradually. In the meantime, in the training of nurses in the field of mental handicap, increased emphasis should be placed on the social aspects of care' (HMSO 1972: paras 557–65, and recommendation 74). This line of thinking was pursued to its logical conclusion by the Jay Committee of Enquiry into Mental Handicap Nursing and Care (HMSO 1979), which envisaged a service based on small local residential units staffed by a new class of 'care workers' certified by the Central Council for Education and Training in Social Work. In effect, nursing was invited to abandon the territory awarded to it in 1919 in favour of social work.

Such a development is less radical than it might seem in the context of the history of developments in health visiting, which will be discussed in Chapter 9, where there has been a similar loss of work to local authority social services over the last half century. There are also precedents for the fission of nursing to create new paramedical occupations with more specialized functions and skills, from physiotherapy and radiography earlier in the century to ODA attendants in the 1980s. On this occasion, however, the proposal aroused considerable resistance for reasons which remain to be explained in full. The various nursing organizations produced rival plans for reshaping the education and role of nurses for the mentally handicapped (Jaehnig 1979, Ryan with Thomas 1980: 135–52). Their training was substantially modified along these lines in 1981, although both the nursing and social work press continue to show evidence of conflict between the two occupations over the ownership of territory in the new region of facilities that are developing for this client group.

Mental nurses have been less directly threatened from outside the occupation. Indeed, the revival of interest in organic treatments, with the continuing development of psychoactive drugs, may even serve to consolidate their position. But they clearly remain under pressure from assimilationists in general nursing. The Briggs Report had proposed to deal with mental nursing as a specialism to be entered after a general 18-month foundation course, reviving models from the 1920s, while the General Nursing Council (1978) *Statement of Educational Policy* reasserted the desirability of eight to twelve weeks' general training for mental nurses.

The reluctant partner

As with any other historical inquiry, the conclusions which can be drawn from the history of mental nursing depend upon the questions which were asked at the beginning. If the investigator starts from questions of education, technical standards, or professional status, it is not difficult to use the official or semi-official publications of the occupation to create an impression of steady incremental improvement. The increasingly secure scientific basis of therapy is seen as the source of more effective care leading to better quality training and a higher status for mental nurses. Each forward step is marked by the announcement of the death of custodial attitudes and behaviour.

If one concentrates on the average experience of the average patient in the average institution, it emerges that custodial habits have a way of clinging rather tenaciously to life. Some of this reflects the enduring poverty of the system. Indeed it is arguable that the resources available have been in constant decline since the great wave of Victorian public investment in county asylums. The NHS did little to inject much-needed resources into the system. While the NHS made consultant psychiatric provision more widely available it fragmented the administration of the services and gave them the lowest priority for its inadequate investment capital. Successive management reorganizations have merely shuffled the pieces on the board to conceal the long-standing attempts of governments of all parties to run the NHS on a level of expenditure well below that of our major Western European neighbours. The consequences for mental nursing were spelt out by Sir Aubrey Lewis in 1949:

> The position is so ominous that palliative measures, desirable in themselves, are likely to be of little use. The process of determination in numbers has gone so far, that it will now operate to further the declension, since depleted staff in every grade means more arduous and less satisfying work, longer hours, and less stimulus for those who remain; the deterrent effect of this upon student recruits and potential recruits is obvious. (DHSS 94198/4/2A)

That verdict might have been passed at any time in the present century.

The fortunes of mental nursing have been intimately linked to those of the mental sector as a whole. As an occupation, mental nursing was a somewhat arbitrary creation of the Victorian lunacy legislation which swept up a miscellaneous collection of sick and deviant people and planted them in asylums rather than in prisons or workhouses. The medicalization of the asylums, and their ultimate reconceptualization as hospitals, reconstituted custodial attendants as nurses for the mentally sick and the defective. But the separation between the asylums and both the voluntary hospitals and the Poor Law infirmaries meant that the prospects for occupational unification were limited. General nursing and the nursing of the mentally disordered could be linked only to the extent that mental illness was defined as essentially organic and that psychiatrists accepted the model of general medicine. Otherwise, the doctors would demand a more specialized helper and the general nurses would resist the theoretical dilution of their occupational knowledge, exemplified by the opposition to the incorporation of mental deficiency nursing under the GNC in 1919. The result was the uneasy co-existence of the RMPA and the GNC as rival certifying bodies for more than thirty years.

The break-up of unified administrative arrangements for mental health service under the NHS created the conditions for the fusion of mental nursing into a unified nursing occupation. This was reinforced by the growth of effective physical treatments in psychiatry. It was no longer necessary to impose a general curriculum on mental nursing, except in so far as it was thought essential to the creation of a common occupational culture, because psychiatry now demanded a biomedical foundation for its helpers' work.

With the questioning of institutional care since the early 1960s, however, mental nursing has experienced a crisis of occupational identity, which has left it exposed to encroachment from two directions. One is the growth of social work and social work-controlled care assistants, and of psychological therapists both inside and outside the health service. Despite the changes forced on nursing by its response to the Jay Report, it has continued to lose ground. The other is the continuing pressure towards assimilation reflected in the Briggs Report and, as Chapter 10 discusses, persisting in the Project 2000 debates. Proposals for reforms in nurse training are based on the assumption that there is indeed a common core to nursing work and that mental nursing can be treated as a post-basic specialty, on the model of medical education. The nursing process has been urged on the psychiatric sector as a method of nursing practice, again largely in the interest of creating a common language and culture. But, as indicated above, this unity is a fragile creation of recent historical origin. It remains vulnerable to the long-term shift from health to social services which is discussed below. There seems little prospect of a divorce between the reluctant spouses of general and mental nursing but it would be unwise to dismiss the possibility of a continuing decline in the role of nursing within the psychiatric services if the model imposed by the stronger partner proves too inflexible for the changing circumstances of the late twentieth century.

Chapter eight

Midwifery

Most of this book has been about nursing in institutions. This is an appropriate emphasis for a study of the development of the modern occupation which is so dominated by the experience of hospital work and the sheer numbers of active registered nurses employed in it. But we must keep its historical place in proportion. At the outset we stressed that most nursing work in the nineteenth century, as always, would have been performed by other members of the sick person's household. The poor might engage a handywoman of their own class to assist while the better-off hired a private nurse to supplement their other servants. Both types of care provider became more or less extinct during the inter-war period. This chapter and the next will attempt to account for their decline and to examine how the social space which they vacated was colonized and redefined as part of the domain of the official occupation of nursing. In present day terms, we shall be considering the work of midwives, health visitors and district nurses, although it is important not to impose these categories uncritically onto the historical record. Each of these specialties has tended to be the subject of separate studies, often for the purpose of constructing a distinctive official history and furthering sectional claims to particular elements of their common work. The result is a literature which substantially overstates their differences.

For the purpose of exposition, we shall have to divide our own account, concentrating on midwifery in this chapter and the other types of home nursing in the next. Before embarking on this, however, it is essential to balance the division by signalling their common features. As we shall show, all three of these specialties exemplify the same conflict between attempts to create 'new professions' for middle- or upper-class women and to co-opt the handywoman class in the moral regulation of the sick and their

145

families. But there were also changes in the social and technical context of home care which bore upon all three.

Home nursing and social change

We have already drawn attention to the extent to which changes in both general and mental nursing were driven by changes in the technology of medicine. Whatever its claims to a distinctive contribution to the division of labour in health care, hospital nursing was also a form of dilution which allowed doctors' skills to be reserved for more sophisticated tasks, however these were then defined. In the process nurses took over work from the treatment assistants described in Chapter 1. Given that the middle and upper classes made little use of the hospitals, though, the latter part of the nineteenth century saw a widening gap between the support available to doctors in their home and their hospital practices. Previous writers (e.g. Carpenter 1977a, 1977b, Gamarnikow 1978) have remarked on the likeness between the hospitals and the Victorian household with the patriarchal doctor being assisted by the lady matron organizing the nurse servants. But the converse is equally important: as the nurse servants acquired more technical skills, home care could achieve parity only with that available in hospital by recruiting people with comparable training. This is the other side of much of the earlier discussion of the economic basis of the sisterhoods (pp. 28–9), the raising of capital for the modernization of hospital training (p. 60), the demand met by hospitals renting out their staff for private work (pp. 59–60) and the consumer support for registration (pp. 79–80).

By the end of the First World War, residential domestic servants had disappeared from all but the richest households and never returned. Without other servants the private nurse could not maintain a distinctive identity as a specialist. The middle classes also seem to have started occupying smaller houses with no space for the nurse to live in. If continuous attention were needed, the patient would have to go to the nurse rather than vice versa. Something like this may lie behind the rise of the nursing homes, which continued during the 1920s. Between the 1921 and 1931 censuses, the number of patients in these institutions increased from 25,981 to 54,290 (Abel-Smith 1960: 128).[1]

Even if staff with appropriate skills could be recruited, both home nursing and nursing homes found it difficult to match the physical facilities of the major voluntary hospitals. Post-war practice demanded large and cumbersome equipment, like X-ray machines, and specialized environments, like operating theatres, which were costly to provide and maintain. These spread into the larger Poor Law infirmaries in urban areas which were increasingly involved in acute medicine. By 1929, when the Poor Law was finally absorbed by local government, many of these institutions were virtually indistinguishable from voluntary hospitals in their facilities and case mix, although their staffing levels still tended to be lower (Crowther 1981: 182–90, Stevens 1966: 59).[2]

If these changes were pulling patients of all classes towards official health care provision, many of the previous barriers to access were also being lowered. Poor Law reform had removed the legal disadvantages of pauperization from the sick poor, although the social stigma of the workhouse and its infirmary lingered for many years. Working-class patients in regular employment, mostly skilled men, were covered by the National Insurance scheme set up under an act of 1911. With subsequent extensions, this embraced 40 per cent of the population by 1938 (Stevens 1966: 53). Although it paid for only general practitioner care, the terms of the scheme encouraged GPs to refer cases on to hospital-based specialists and its administration provided a model for the growth of private insurance. By 1935, 25 per cent of the population had some coverage for hospital expenses and more than half the total revenue of the voluntary hospitals came from their charges to private patients (Stevens 1966; 59). The Radcliffe Infirmary in Oxford, for example, derived 70 per cent of its income from a weekly contribution scheme. The main exclusion from these developments was maternity care, although some local authorities made generous use of the powers which they acquired during the 1920s and 1930s to provide free or heavily subsidized services.

Home nursing was also affected by demographic and epidemiological change. Improvements in diet, housing and sanitation led to a dramatic decline in the incidence of infectious diseases (McKeown 1965: 39–58, Winter 1982: 100–20). The consequent improvements in both adult and child mortality rates had not yet worked through to create a large population of elderly people who might need continuing nursing care. In 1901, 4.7 per cent of the UK population were over 65. This rose to 7.5 per cent by 1931 but was still well short of the 1985 level of 15 per cent (Central Statistical Office 1987: Table 2.3). The birth rate declined steadily from 1880 to 1940 with the exception of a brief post-war rise between 1920 and 1925 (Macfarlane and Mugford 1984: Table A3.1. See Table 3 on p. 148).

This was reflected in family size: 70 per cent of couples who married in the 1870s had four or more children while 70 per cent of those marrying in the 1920s had three or fewer (Wrigley 1969: 185–

Table 3 Fertility Rate: England and Wales 1838–1981

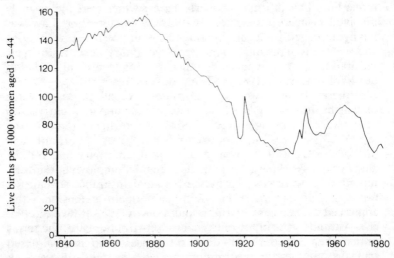

Source: Macfarlane and Mugford (1984: 28)

91). There were fewer babies to generate demand for midwifery and post-partum care and fewer conflicting calls on a caregiver trying to nurse a sick member of the household.

These developments did not have a uniform impact. In particular, in many rural areas and some traditional working-class communities, there seems every reason to suppose that handy-women continued to play a significant role in health care until the arrival of the NHS or even beyond. Nevertheless, the combined impact of cultural, economic and technological change radically altered the terms of the competition between official and irregular nurses and, arguably, led to a substantial absolute contraction in the demand for home care. The decline of the irregular nurse, however, was not solely the result of these environmental changes but also reflected the growing power of their official competitors.

The first of these official competitors to be considered here will be the midwives. Their relationship with general nursing has been an ambivalent one. Although most contemporary midwives have had an initial training in general nursing, there is a tendency to regard this linkage as some sort of historical accident and to insist on the distinctiveness of midwifery as an occupation. This reflects the extent to which modern nursing is an imperfect fusion of different areas of caring work as outlined in Chapter 1. Midwifery was the first of these to establish a legal definition of its membership and their activities. Indeed it was able to achieve a monopoly of practice, backed by law, which other branches of nursing have never been able to achieve.[3] Nevertheless, midwifery has been shaped by many of the same influences as general nursing and riven by the same tension between the creation of an independent profession for women and the provision of skilled auxiliaries for doctors. Its absorption into the regulatory structure represented by the UKCC, however, provides at least a minimal justification for considering it as part of the occupation of nursing.

Midwifery before 1800

Just as with general nursing, midwifery was practised in the early nineteenth century by a great variety of men and women with a range of skills and experiences. Sarah Gamp advertised herself as a midwife as much as a nurse. But any assessment of the picture is complicated by the economic rivalries between the various types of practitioner involved. Most of the portraits of handywomen midwives as drunken hags come either from doctors or, later, from the would-be lady practitioners. They can be matched by the image of man-midwives as meddlesome perverts contributed by literate women and genteel men.

Few of the female midwives in this period would have been full-time practitioners. They varied in skill and status from the village handywoman, combining midwifery with her other trades, to marginal members of the middle classes. In the early nineteenth century, the former mostly delivered other poor women for a fee which was unlikely to exceed 2s 6d and also covered help around the home for a few days after the birth. Indeed, there might not even be a cash transaction involved at all, but an exchange of goods or a promise of future services in kind. For these women midwifery and other handywoman activities are probably best understood as informal work, an interlude between cleaning or laundering or other casual female employment. Some of them might also be engaged by charities or by the Poor Law, which Donnison (1977: 59) suggests could give them greater recognition and attract a better class of patient. None of these women were likely to have received any sort of training except that those assisting Poor Law medical officers or seeing patients referred by a local doctor, because they could not afford his fees, might have been given some sort of instruction on an individual basis (Donnison 1977: 60).

In the larger towns and cities, salaried midwives could be found in some hospitals and infirmaries. They were paid £30–£40 per year, about the same as an upper servant or a governess. Others mixed contract work for charitable foundations with private practice and could earn as much as a skilled worker or an elementary schoolteacher. A few could expect to be engaged by wealthy women who particularly wanted a female attendant, when their fees might go as high as thirty guineas per delivery. This group were the most likely to have received some sort of instruction, usually at one of the few lying-in hospitals or dispensaries, which were the only parts of the voluntary sector to accept maternity cases (Smith 1979: 45, Donnison 1977: 60). Smith (1979: 41) also cites some examples of middle-class midwives in Bristol with a practice among wealthy radical families, who appear to have learnt their skills from a medically qualified male relative.

Female midwifery was a low-technology craft with little use of instruments. Patients supplied their own linen, utensils and drugs. This probably reduced the risk of cross-infection, but it limited the resources available to the midwife in difficult cases. For a normal delivery, the reliance on manual skills and dexterity may have made for safer practice than the use of instruments by a busy doctor anxious to accelerate the process so that he could go on to the next case. But if anything went wrong the consequences could be serious. Smith (1979: 42–4) quotes several examples, including that of Mary H. from St Marylebone in London in 1840. She was in labour for 17 hours with her ninth child but the midwife refused to call a surgeon. The baby was delivered alive after a labour of 26 hours and Mary H. then died of exhaustion. The midwife failed to get the placenta out because it broke while she was pulling at it. A post-mortem examination found the whole body 'bloodless and flaccid'.

As various references have already suggested, it is important to remember that the medical profession already had a well-established role in midwifery work. Before the 1730s, the involvement of official medicine in midwifery was limited to the employment of a surgeon in abnormal labours, mostly to destroy the infant by performing a craniotomy. But, since the 1750s, the surgeon–apothecaries had steadily expanded their practice in this area. They had gradually become accepted as the proper attendants for any complicated labour and for such normal labours as women were willing or able to pay their fees (Loudon 1986: 6–7).

The extent of the doctors' skills should not be underestimated. The economic importance of midwifery to general practice gave them a considerable incentive to develop their knowledge and techniques. Private courses in midwifery for medical practitioners began to develop during the second half of the eighteenth century and were readily available to most students intending to set up in general practice by 1800. These included experience of deliveries both in hospital and in homes in the surrounding district. They did not form part of the official curriculum of the medical schools but were taught by men affiliated to them as lecturers in midwifery (Loudon 1986: 7, forthcoming).

In elite circles, however, midwifery or obstetrics was regarded as a socially disreputable specialty. At Edinburgh University. which tended to follow Continental practice and was a pioneer of obstetric teaching for medical students, James Hamilton, Professor of Midwifery from 1800 to 1839, found his wife snubbed at a charity ball as 'unfit company for respectable ladies and gentlemen' (Donnison 1977: 43). In London, both the Royal Colleges, of Physicians and of Surgeons, excluded practitioners of midwifery from their Fellowships and, hence, from any access to office or power. After the Apothecaries Act 1815 the medical colleges strengthened their control over the curriculum and imposed their prejudices about the fitness of midwifery as work for a gentleman. The shift of power from patients to the professional elite reduced the competitive pressure to acquire midwifery skills. Contemporaries clearly recognized a decline in the standards of medical practice in this area which was not fully remedied until midwifery became a mandatory part of basic medical education in 1879.

There are suggestions, however, that the situation did begin to improve from the late 1820s. The surgeons included questions about midwifery in their examinations, although they were not compulsory and the University of London set a paper on midwifery when it began to offer the MB degree in the 1840s. Male students took over such opportunities as there were for learning on the wards of the lying-in hospitals. The British Lying-In Hospital in London, for instance, admitted male students in 1831 and within ten years was training as many of them as it was female midwives (Donnison 1977: 53). This, in effect, was the counterpart of the informal improvements in general nursing before 1850, except that it was focused on medical practitioners.

As in other areas of medical work, the gradual consolidation of knowledge and technique generated a demand for a reliable person to relieve the doctor of the labour-intensive task of monitoring his patient's condition. In this case, the doctor's involvement could be reserved for the risky business of the delivery, rather than being absorbed in, for example, inactive sitting with a labouring woman. The British Lying-In Hospital began courses in 1826 for monthly nurses to assist medical attendants in labour and to provide some post-partum care. By the

1840s, it was training three times as many of these women as it was midwives (Donnison 1977: 53).

As with midwives, it is not difficult to find horrifying stories of medical attendance in childbirth and Smith (1979: 24–6) gives some gruesome examples. One relates to William Gaches, a Norfolk apothecary, delivering a woman of her tenth child in 1845.

> The child was born after a labour of many hours; the mother was screaming with agony as Gaches thrust repeatedly in her womb for the delayed afterbirth. At last he pulled out 'something' which he hid from the midwife assisting him. The post-mortem showed that he had pulled out several pounds of womb and small intestine. (Smith 1979: 25)

If the labour did present problems, though, the doctor had few resources available: tincture of ergot for haemorrhage; tincture of digitalis or bleeding for the expulsion of the placenta; tincture of cannabis indicus as a pain reliever. Chloroform did not become available until 1847 and took some years to come into widespread use (Smith 1979: 17). Forceps became known during the second half of the eighteenth century but were rarely employed (Loudon 1986: 18–19). For all this a general practitioner might expect a fee of three to four guineas by the middle of the nineteenth century, with about a quarter going to any midwife or nurse who had assisted him (Smith 1979: 27).

Neither midwives nor doctors had much involvement with a woman's care outside the immediate period of her confinement until the twentieth century. The actual diagnosis of pregnancy was something of an art. Although fetal heart sounds were identified on the Continent in the early 1820s, and the stethoscope used to monitor them, this had little place in British practice till the late 1830s (Smith 1979: 16–17, Oakley 1984: 25–6). The main technique employed was manual examination, which could yield reliable results for a skilled practitioner. Nevertheless, the records of hospitals for women's disorders in the 1860s suggest that even specialists could find themselves operating on a pregnant woman in the belief that she had some kind of uterine growth (Moscucci 1984).[4] Ante-natal care, then, generally consisted of little more than advice on diet, rest and personal conduct, derived from the idiosyncratic theories of the practitioner. It was not an essential element of the package. Similarly, a doctor or midwife would normally cease to be involved in care about ten days after delivery, although a family might employ a monthly nurse for somewhat longer.

The division of the market between doctors and midwives varied from one part of the country to another. In the 1840s, it was acknowledged that many women were still giving birth without the presence of an attendant who would claim any particular skill, even to the extent of being described as a 'village midwife'. A completely free choice was available only to those women who could pay the fees and who lived in an area with a population sufficiently affluent to support a variety of practitioners. Other women were obliged to accept whatever practitioner, doctor or midwife, lying-in charities or the Poor Law would provide. Estimates from the 1870s suggest that midwives had the larger share of the market. Nationally, they were thought to attend 70 per cent of all births (Donnison 1977: 77). They handled somewhat more work in rural areas and among the poor in industrial towns: general practitioners had more business in market towns and in the more affluent parts of London and its suburbs (Loudon 1986: 9). Cost and access barriers meant that medical attendance on a normal delivery was largely, although not exclusively, a middle-class phenomenon.

It should not be thought that the results of this pattern of maternity care were regarded as satisfactory by contemporaries. William Farr, the Statistical Superintendent of the Registrar-General's Office, persistently denounced the maternal mortality rate in his annual reports from 1841 onwards (Donnison 1977: 53, Loudon 1986). The official statistics showed a rate of six maternal deaths per thousand registered births in the 1840s, although the reliability of these figures is somewhat questionable. More reliable data became available from the 1850s and these place the rate at 4.9 per thousand births within a range of 3.8 to 5.4 per thousand which remained unchanged until the late 1930s (Loudon 1986: 3).[5] Farr drew attention to the initiatives of other European governments, particularly in the training of midwives which he regarded as making a significant contribution to their superior maternal mortality rates. In fact, the picture is somewhat more complicated because of different systems of recording and mixes of provision. Comparing figures from 17 European lying-in hospitals between 1840 and 1870, Loudon (forthcoming) found maternal mortality rates ranging from 9 to 156 per thousand births with the main British institutions towards the lower end. Despite Farr's enthusiasm, however, there was no real consensus that the education of midwives was the best way forward. The following decade saw a number of experiments and much competition between the advocates of midwifery and those who favoured the improvement of medical care, possibly by the training and selective involvement of women doctors.

The search for improvement

The movement towards the licensing of midwifery reflects a complex mixture of motives, objectives and sectional interests. It has been examined in detail by Donnison (1977). From her account, it is possible to identify five different groups, each of which had its own distinct agenda.

The first of these was initially organized around the Female Medical Society, founded in 1862 to press for the admission of women to the medical profession. They saw midwifery as a high-status occupation for educated women working in parallel with male doctors across the whole range of patients and obstetric conditions. There was some internal difference of emphasis upon whether this was better achieved by setting up a distinct occupation from medicine with its own licensing arrangements, or possibly subject to the authority of the General Medical Council, or by getting women accepted for medical qualification in the expectation that they would choose to concentrate on this area of practice. As the barriers to women entering the medical profession were reduced in the 1870s and 1880s, this group dissolved, although the former idea was kept alive by other organizations like the Obstetrical Association of Midwives and the Matrons' Aid Society. Their programme eventually attracted the qualified support of Florence Nightingale who saw in it an ideal quite different from that of general nursing and an aspiration preferable to that of women competing with men inside the medical profession.

Miss Nightingale herself was more closely identified with a second group of reformers whose prime interest was in the provision of better maternity care for the poor and saw the midwife as a low-cost alternative to doctors. Donnison fails to recognize this because of her reliance on the traditional picture of Nightingale nursing. Baly (1986: 65–81) shows that the short-lived scheme at King's College for the training of 'midwifery nurses' was very much directed at producing all-purpose obstetric practitioners to work in poor rural parishes. The women involved seem to have been recruited mainly through local clergy or missionary associations and lived under the rules of the St John Sisterhood. Baly estimates that the scheme produced about 40 midwives over a five-year period, although very little is known about them. The scheme is usually said to have collapsed because of an outbreak of puerperal fever. In fact, Baly shows that the death rate was not exceptional for English lying-in institutions and argues that it is more plausibly explained by the resignation of Mary Jones, the superintendent, after a dispute with the hospital governors over her High Church enthusiasm. Miss Nightingale's active support for Miss Jones led to a breakdown in relations and the withdrawal of the Nightingale Fund's sponsorship. Although she hoped to revive the scheme elsewhere, the fund's resources were so drained by its contract with St Thomas's that this was never possible.

Although the Local Government Board's president, James Stansfield, expressed some interest in the licensing of midwives in correspondence with the GMC in 1873 and received a deputation from the Midwives' Association, the board seems to have taken no part in the debate until the government finally became committed to backing private members' initiatives for legislation in 1900. Even then it was defined as a public health matter for local authorities rather than as a concern for the Poor Law. The board's silence on the question of midwives may, however, simply reflect a greater emphasis on the better provision of care under the Poor Law by doctors, which Donnison does not acknowledge. Hodgkinson (1967: 549) points out that medical supervision became available more readily where resident medical officers were appointed to the new generation of infirmaries from the 1860s. Poor Law medical officers could be cruelly overworked. In Bethnal Green, Dr Defriez was dealing with 100 midwifery cases per year on top of 60 acute surgical cases and 40–80 home visits for minor ailments. Similarly, parish midwives were recorded as claiming for up to 600 deliveries in a year (Smith 1979: 53). These midwives probably varied as much in quality as before 1850. In some areas, like Liverpool and Brighton, there were well-developed training schemes and low maternal death rates. In others, guardians still patronized the village handywoman at 3d a time.

The third and fourth factions both drew their main support from within the medical profession. The specialists in the Obstetrical Society, which had been formed in 1858, saw licensing as a way of establishing a second-tier practitioner to relieve them of unprofitable routine work and to by-pass the general practitioners. The GPs represented by the BMA saw licensing as a device for controlling or supressing cut-price competitors. It is difficult to disentangle the elements of self-interest and public good in their cases. Both groups saw the midwife as a woman of relatively humble origins providing a basic service to mothers of her own class at a price they could afford. The doctors would secure a monopoly in the treatment of better-off patients but poor women should receive more competent and sanitary care. This was not a trivial matter. As with district nursing, there were serious doubts about whether lady midwives would be willing to work in poor areas for the fees available. Even those with a missionary zeal or private means might be reluctant to bury themselves in remote parts of the country for any length of time. If the standards of midwifery were set too high, unlicensed practice was bound to persist.

Finally, mention must be made of the lady nurses organized in the British Nurses' Association under the leadership of Mrs Bedford Fenwick. Displaying her characteristic opportunism, she wanted to use midwifery licensing as a stalking horse in the campaign for the registration of general nurses. However, an alliance proposed in 1888 with the Matrons' Aid Society, now renamed the Midwives' Institute, was firmly rebuffed. Both groups were recruiting a similar type of woman with some cross-membership and they shared a common strategy of co-operating with sections of the medical profession. But the Midwives' Institute insisted that their members were independent practitioners rather than medical auxiliaries. As such they required separate and prior consideration. The BMA retained its interest and continued to agitate for midwife registration but the institute had established much better political connections and played a larger part in the push for legislation.

Donnison's work lies within a particular tradition in the study of occupational development which tends to emphasize the role of 'demand' factors in the establishment of professional licensing. This emphasizes the role of pressure groups which succeed by either political skill, economic power or moral force in persuading policymakers or legislators to accede to their demands. It is probably for this reason that so much of her attention is focused on the activities of well-connected ladies and their medical friends or rivals. But there are two other factors in the situation which are also important. One is the attitude of clients or patients and the other is the attitude of the state. It is no use passing licensing laws if the public will not use the service and modern governments are not notably enthusiastic about creating artificial monopolies (Dingwall and Fenn 1987).

These debates may have aroused great passions among a literate elite, which wished to impose its own view of progress. They were, however, almost wholly irrelevant to most women. Whether on grounds of price, skill, availability or custom, traditional midwives were the practitioners chosen for the majority of births. In many communities they continued to serve the poor well into the twentieth century. This was not purely the result of their inexpensiveness compared with midwives registered under the

1902 Act but because of their willingness to provide additional domestic services or to follow local preferences about childbirth rituals. The fishing community in Aberdeen, for instance, had a traditional practitioner who was still doing deliveries in the 1940s and regularly consulted until her death in the 1960s.

Those women who were, increasingly, choosing doctors to attend them had good reason to do so. Although the subject was still disclaimed by the ancient English universities and the Royal Colleges, medical education in midwifery improved considerably after 1870 (Smith 1979: 23–4). The main problem was the difficulty of giving students practical experience because of the limited number of hospital births. In 1890 only 0.3 per cent of births occurred in voluntary hospitals with another 1 per cent in Poor Law infirmaries, which were not used for teaching. The majority of births did not take place in hospital until 1946 (Loudon 1986: 22). Nevertheless, doctors were developing a few important techniques, especially in the use of chloroform as a pain reliever, which made their services more attractive to women. Those mothers who were rich enough to afford the choice do not seem to have considered that nature assisted by a midwife was overwhelmingly preferable to a pleasant haze of anaesthesia and a pain-free delivery. Midwives might be licensed but women could not be compelled to engage their services where they had the means to choose.[6]

Donnison (1977: 167) notes, rather in passing, the shift in the political climate by 1902 and the military confusion of the Boer War. This was a critical moment in the development of health visiting but is of limited relevance to midwifery. The debate on the Midwives Bill opened in the middle of the furore over General J. F. Maurice's public criticism of the physical condition of recruits to the army and his claim that the cause lay in the poor provision made for maternal and child welfare. But the measure was already assured of government support by this point and its drafting reflected agreement by the Home Office, the Local Government Board and the Privy Council. Indeed, this coalition made it possible to stiffen the terms of the bill over the objections of medical interests and to establish the Central Midwives Board as a body directly accountable to the Privy Council rather than being subordinated to the GMC. The National Efficiency debate launched by Maurice's article undoubtedly facilitated the bill's passage but it seems an implausible cause. The exact reasons for the government's change of heart between 1898, when the President of the Council refused to support the bill because of medical opposition, and 1900, when he authorized his staff to help draft the legislation, remain obscure. It is clear, however, that the government was not willing to abandon midwifery registration to the medical profession but considered that it was of sufficient policy importance to require a separate, publicly accountable system of licensing (Donnison 1977: 169). This suggests that the shift in policy should be seen alongside other attempts to improve public health provision in the late 1890s, as in the renewed pressure from the LGB to raise standards of general nursing in the Poor Law Infirmaries (pp. 67–8) and the strengthening of the Infant Life Preservation Act to regulate fostering and child minding (p. 183), rather than as the first of the welfare reforms of the Edwardian era. The enthusiasm with which it was implemented, however, certainly reflects the stimulation of the social programme of the 1906–11 Liberal Government.

An independent practitioner?

The Central Midwives Board began its work in December 1902. It had nine members, four medical practitioners nominated by the Royal Colleges of Physicians and Surgeons, the Society of Apothecaries and the Midwives' Institute, two members, one of whom had to be a woman, nominated by the Privy Council, and one member each nominated by the Association of County Councils, Queen Victoria's Jubilee Institute for Nurses and the Royal British Nurses' Association. There was no statutory obligation to appoint a midwife, although the Privy Council, the Queen's Institute and the RBNA all used their powers to nominate prominent members of the Midwives' Institute. This resulted in a board which, unusually for its time, comprised six men and three women. Its jurisdiction was restricted to England and Wales.

The board's first act was to set up a roll of practising midwives. The legislation permitted any woman who had been in *bona fide* practice for one year and was of good character to apply for registration. This window would be open until April 1905. From that date no woman would be allowed to use the title of 'midwife' unless she were registered under the act and from April 1910 no woman would be able 'habitually and for gain' to attend women in childbirth unless she were registered or working under a doctor's supervision.

The results surprised, even shocked, contemporaries. The 1891 census had identified about 3,000 midwives although this was generally acknowledged to be an underestimate because of the extent of part-time practice. J. H. Aveling, one of the leaders of the Obstetrical Society, had thought there might be 9,000 women doing this work. Other estimates ranged up to 15,000 (Donnison 1977: 218–19) but when the CMB Roll closed, it contained 22,308 names. Less than half of these (9,787) had any recognizable certificate in midwifery. The principal qualification, held by 7,465 women, was the licence awarded by the Obstetrical Society of London (LGB 1914–15: 68). Many of this group, however, were trained nurses who were not practising as midwives but wanted to be on the roll in order to keep open their career options. As a result, the *bona fide* midwives were an even more important source of attendants in childbirth than the simple figures might suggest (Cowell and Wainwright 1981: 42).

The supervision of midwives was delegated to county councils and county boroughs. Local authorities varied greatly in the enthusiasm with which they took on this duty and the use they made of their powers. Their initial surveys revealed a discouraging picture of the skill and availability of midwives. In Worcestershire, 581 midwives registered and notified the local authority of their intention to practise. Only 4 per cent had any sort of certificate, 11 per cent were illiterate, 17 per cent were over the age of 65, 8 per cent were rated 'very dirty', 16 per cent had no washable dresses, 10 per cent lived in 'filthy' houses and 5 per cent were suspected of being heavy drinkers. The Medical Officer of Health for the West Riding of Yorkshire reckoned that 37 per cent of his midwives were illiterate. In Liverpool, on the other hand, which had an active tradition of public health work and a vigorous District Nursing Association, 70 per cent of the midwives had been trained at the local lying-in hospital while many of the remainder held the Obstetrical Society's Certificate (Towler and Bramall 1986: 190). Durham reported 264 notified midwives, of whom 20 per cent had some training, while Norfolk had just 70 midwives of whom 14 per cent were trained (Cowell and Wainwright 1981: 46). These traditional practitioners inevitably played an important part in the supply of midwifery services. Even in a county borough like Rotherham, which had made a particular effort to implement the 1902 Act, certified midwives were thought to be dealing with only about half the deliveries (Smith 1979: 57).

The CMB, then, faced action on two fronts: the upgrading of standards among existing practitioners and the development of training programmes to certify new entrants. But the first of these responsibilities was exercised at one remove by the local authorities who were immediately responsible for the supervision of midwives and had the power to suspend them from practice, although not to withdraw their licence. This power had originally been intended as a measure against cross-infection but this restriction was deleted during the bill's passage through parliament. Consequently, in the hands of unsympathetic supervisors, it could be used to harass midwives and protect the general practitioners' share of deliveries in a neighbourhood. Both areas of initiative were also constrained by the limits of available resources and by the need to preserve access to some sort of maternity service throughout the whole country.

It is difficult to establish just how much use was made by local authorities of their supervising powers. The CMB itself complained in 1909 and 1910 of the difficulty of getting statistical returns and took this as evidence of a lack of energy in the administration of the act. The 1910 report mentions 53 cases of 'malpractice, negligence and misconduct' reported to the local supervising authorities (Towler and Bramall 1986: 193) and, in the same year, 103 cases were heard by the board (Lewis 1980: 144). Sixty of these led to removal from the roll (Cowell and Wainwright 1981: 46). The picture is further complicated by 'voluntary' deregistrations. Eighty-eight women withdrew from the roll in 1910. We have no way of knowing to what extent these reflect supervisors' pressures or a recognition by the women themselves that they could not meet the standards prescribed by CMB rules. There is little evidence of any systematic attempts at in-service education. The Midwives' Institute ran some lectures and encouraged the formation of local associations, while some supervising authorities also seem to have organized classes.

More effort appears to have been focused on the accreditation of hospitals to offer training courses. Approved institutions could offer a three-month programme as preparation for the examinations organized quarterly by the board. These consisted of a three-hour written paper and a fifteen-minute oral examination. However, the exercise of these powers by the CMB rapidly brought it into conflict with the Local Government Board. Although only about 1.3 per cent of all births took place in institutions, the bulk of these occurred in Poor Law infirmaries. The Midwives' Act 1902 had the effect of requiring that these births would either have to be supervised by a doctor or conducted by a licensed midwife. It was, therefore, of some importance to the infirmaries that they could train their own staff. Rightly or wrongly, the CMB was perceived to be dominated by voluntary hospital interests and the infirmaries felt that their applications for accreditation were being deliberately delayed and then treated more critically than those from the voluntary sector. The LGB were also concerned that the CMB's system of inspection could act in opposition to the work of their own inspectorate. Here, too, then, the CMB's aspirations were tempered by political anxieties about access to services. While it might be possible to set a high standard in the densely provided London area, this would denude the rest of the country. In 1907, the Privy Council agreed to exempt Poor Law infirmaries from the CMB's accreditation arrangements, although their students would still have to pass the CMB examinations (White 1978: 90–2). This exemption lasted until 1924, by which time the Ministry of Health, which inherited many of the LGB's functions in 1919, had taken a firmer grip on the CMB's membership (Donnison, 1977: 192–3).

The concern over access was also responsible for one minor breach in the legal restrictions on unlicensed practice. From April 1910, no one would be allowed to attend women in childbirth 'habitually and for gain' other than a licensed midwife or under the supervision of a doctor. As this date approached, a certain amount of agitation developed around the country among unregistered midwives who faced exclusion from practice. Eventually, the CMB responded by agreeing to license another 515 *bona fide* midwives on the recommendation of local authorities (Cowell and Wainwright 1981: 45, 47).

Of much greater significance, though, was the difficulty of enforcing the 'habitually and for gain' prohibition in the face of opposition from the medical profession and patients, who colluded to perpetuate the practice of 'handywomen' well into the 1930s. The declining birth rate and relatively open market forced general practitioners and midwives into a competition which caused considerable suffering to patients. Midwives could undercut GPs on fees for normal deliveries but were required by CMB rules to summon a doctor if complications developed. A midwife might be reluctant to lose her fee and the confidence of clients by sending for help and a GP might delay his response as a means of signalling to potential customers that they were better advised to book him in the first place. Moreover, if the family could only afford a midwife, he could not be sure of receiving his fee. A midwife might find herself obliged to guarantee this personally, until 1919 when local authorities were required to pay and then try to recover their costs from the family. If the midwife did not obtain medical assistance, she was in breach of CMB rules and could be disciplined.

Systematic ante-natal care and planning for deliveries did not reach the majority of women until the Second World War (Oakley 1984: 133). Thus most deliveries were, if not emergencies in a clinical sense, only loosely predicted events. Faced with a criminal charge, an unlicensed midwife could claim that she was merely helping out with an unanticipated birth. A bigger loophole was the provision for unlicensed women to work under medical supervision. In practice, this often meant that a general practitioner would agree to sign the relevant forms for notification of the birth and National Insurance claims in return for a share of the fee. If challenged he would claim the woman had been acting as his nurse and he had been unavoidably prevented from attending the delivery. The General Medical Council threatened to discipline doctors who participated in such arrangements in 1916 but they were not substantially eliminated until further legislation in 1926 and 1936 removed the 'habitually and for gain' loophole and required 'maternity nurses' assisting doctors to be qualified (Lewis 1980: 150, Oakley 1984: 108–9, Towler and Bramall 1986: 207–9, 228).

But it is important to remember that this pattern of service would not have persisted without the acquiescence of patients. In many cases, of course, they were too poor to have a choice: handywomen were cheaper than licensed midwives. A proportion of these were covered by combined district nurse/midwives employed by voluntary nursing associations supported by county council grants. But the Ministry of Health investigation of maternal mortality in the Counties, Urban Districts and County Boroughs of Northern England in 1934–5 acknowledged that these failed to reach many rural areas (HMSO 1937: 252). It has also been suggested that handywomen were preferred by working-class women who needed more help than the licensed midwife was willing to give. One of the effects of licensing and the progressive extension of training was the social closure of the occupation to the traditional 'homely' woman. In 1911, 83 per cent of all midwives were married or widowed and 70 per cent were over the age of 45. By 1931, when women with nurse training had to follow a six-month course and those without, a twelve-month course, 52 per cent of midwives were married or widowed and 48 per cent were over 45 years of age. There was virtually no change in the composition of the female workforce between those dates (Lewis 1980: 144–5). These younger, middle-class women were less ready to give general domestic assistance and preferred to concentrate on the actual delivery itself. By 1933, only 4 per cent of practising midwives had had no formal training, compared with 49 per cent in 1916. (Oakley 1984: 108–9).

The midwives had won an important victory when the National Insurance Act 1911 had placed them on an equal footing with doctors receiving maternity benefit payments from those women covered by its provisions and specified that they must have a free choice of practitioner. They also benefited considerably from the diversion of doctors to the armed forces in the First World War which removed potential competitors and allowed the new licensing system a chance to become fully established. The war also precipitated major extensions of maternity and child care services by local authorities which we shall discuss in Chapter 9. The consequences of this for midwives were rather mixed. Although some of their expenses were reimbursed by local authorities and grants made available for training, the increasing development of municipal ante-natal clinics after 1918 tended to enshrine a medically led model of care. Midwives seem to have had relatively little involvement with these (Lewis 1980: 151, Oakley 1984: 59, 113–4). There was, of course, little incentive for an independent midwife to refer her clients, especially as the surveillance at the clinic was likely to divert them into medical hands and lose her their custom. Moreover, both midwives and general practitioners were coming under pressure from the dramatic increase in hospital confinements. By 1927, 15 per cent of deliveries were occurring in hospital, reaching almost 40 per cent by 1940 (Lewis 1980: 120, Loudon 1986).

This process was driven by several forces. One was the greater economic attractiveness of women patients. Once National Insurance coverage was introduced for many working-class women, the voluntary hospitals began to charge for confinements so that these became a source of income rather than a cost (Lewis 1980: 121). The demands for better training of both doctors and midwives also contributed. One of the reasons why medical students still had relatively little experience of obstetrics as late as the 1920s and 1930s was the limited and uneven provision of in-patient facilities where large numbers of normal and abnormal deliveries could be observed or performed. The teaching hospitals began to invest in new maternity beds and to run down their district services (Lewis 1980: 132). But this shift was also a feature of midwifery training. The CMB had originally allowed midwives to undertake this exclusively in domicilary practice, either with a charity or as an apprentice to an independent practitioner. Janet Campbell, later senior medical officer at the Ministry of Health, had urged in a Carnegie Trust Report in 1917 that all midwives should have some hospital experience in the diagnosis and management of delivery complications and midwifery training does seem to have become concentrated into hospitals during the 1920s, although 16 out of 71 accredited programmes still offered no hospital experience in 1923 (Towler and Bramall 1986: 202, 205). This concentration, of course, also introduced another source of competition between midwifery and medicine, over access to deliveries for teaching purposes.

It is, however, also essential to recognize that the move towards hospital deliveries reflected the positive preferences of many individual women. The handover of Poor Law infirmaries to local authorities in 1929, for instance, removed some of the stigma and the remaining access barriers to these facilities. It was quickly followed by a massive upsurge in demand despite the poor facilities on offer (Lewis 1980: 133–4). Municipally owned or subsidized hospitals were responsible for 32 per cent of all deliveries by 1938 (Ferguson and Fitzgerald 1954: 28). There may have been an element of fashion in this movement but there were also genuine reasons why women might choose a hospital confinement. Probably the most important was the readier availability of pain relief. Ann Oakley (1984: 130) implies that this was some sort of artificially stimulated demand, contrasting evidence of working-class women's views of the birth experience in 1915, when it is largely absent, and in 1945, when the unavailability of analgesia was a major complaint in a Mass Observation survey. It seems more plausible, however, to see this as indicating a growing awareness that something could be done to relieve pain: her quotes from the Mass Observation respondents suggest a resentment that rich women could have comfortable labours in hospital while poor women suffered outside. In the 1930s, pain relief in hospital was still not universal, being used in about 60 per cent of deliveries at the Royal Free Hospital in London in 1932, for example (Lewis 1980: 129). But, as late as 1939, only 0.5 per cent of home deliveries by midwives involved the use of analgesia (Lewis 1980: 146).

There is no suggestion that midwives were hostile to the use of pain relievers but the medical profession and the CMB did not consider chloroform safe for their administration and they were only permitted to use 'gas and air' (nitrous oxide) from 1936 (1946 in Scotland) and then under tightly regulated conditions (Oakley 1984: 110). This could be interpreted in two ways. One is to see it as an anti-competitive move by doctors. By denying midwives access to analgesia, and to a range of other drugs, the medical profession made it more difficult for their rivals to offer a genuine alternative as opposed to a second-best service for the poor. The other is to point to the extent to which midwives had already been conceptually assimilated to nursing by the 1930s and to see this as exactly analogous to earlier experiences with new technology like thermometers, stethoscopes or pulse watches. As Hughes (1971: 311–15) observes, one of the fundamental processes of the division of labour in health care is the making of innovations by doctors which, once routinized, are then delegated to nurses or other paramedical occupations.

In the Carnegie Trust Report (1917), Janet Campbell had already referred to the midwife as occupying 'an exceptional position in the nursing profession' (quoted in Towler and Bramall 1986: 201). This attitude was clearly reflected in Ministry of Health and CMB policies during the 1920s and 1930s (Oakley 1984: 110). From 1916 onwards trained nurses were permitted to undertake a shorter midwifery training and this persisted in the revisions of 1924 and 1937 (Oakley 1984: 109). There seems to have been considerable mobility between midwifery and general nursing during this period (Cowell and Wainwright 1981: 51–2). The Departmental Committee on the Training and Employment of Midwives in 1929 repeated the view of midwifery as a 'branch of the nursing profession' and expressed the fear that midwives would return to general nursing if their conditions of work were not improved (Towler and Bramall 1986: 211, 214, 225–6). By 1936 the majority of pupil midwives were registered nurses. Many of these were seeking midwifery as an additional qualification for career reasons rather than with the intention of practising: only about 25 per cent of those passing the CMB Finals went on to work as midwives by the late 1930s (Ferguson and Fitzgerald 1954: 315).

The reasons for the increasing emphasis on the recruitment of registered nurses rather than direct entrants await further investigation. The ministry's statements do, however, suggest that the view of the midwife as an independent practitioner rather than as a medical assistant had limited support outside the occupation from an earlier date than one might suppose. There is no 'Golden Age' of licensed midwifery in Britain. The occupation was kept alive when it died in America by influential patrons. Whereas leaders of American women's health campaigns had concentrated on reforming the medical profession, their counterparts in England had seen the midwife as an alternative (Brickman 1983: 77–8). By the 1920s, their English equivalents were following the same policy. The Women's Co-operative Guild had proposed a national maternity service in 1914 with trained midwives for all: by 1918 they were demanding a doctor to supervise every case (Lewis 1980: 129).

By the 1930s, the independent practitioner, in the true sense of a licensed midwife who made her own living from fee-for-service practice, was a dying breed. With a declining birth rate and a growing movement towards hospital confinements, the market for her skills was contracting sharply. As we show in the next chapter (pp. 193–4) the district nursing associations were in a chronic state of financial crisis. Midwifery was kept alive only by nationalization under the Midwives Act 1936, which set up a salaried service operated, directly or through contracts with the voluntary associations, by local authorities. This development, provoked by the continuing concern for maternal mortality discussed later in the context of health visiting, provided secure employment for midwives and guaranteed access to midwifery services for clients. Independent practitioners could either join the service, receive compensation for surrendering their certificates to practice or try to continue private work in competition with the heavily subsidized public service. By 1942, only about 15 per cent of midwives were still in private practice (Towler and Bramall 1986: 231).

A state midwifery service

The 1936 Act did not provide a free maternity service. Local authorities were expected to charge women wherever they could afford to pay. But it did mark a significant move towards a greater integration of effort. Theoretically, at least, ante-natal care, delivery and post-partum care could all be linked together with each other and with child care and health services. In practice, of course, the energy and efficiency of local authorities varied as much as ever. There were over 400 authorities providing health care services and 188 responsible for midwifery. Both voluntary and municipal hospitals usually ran competing ante-natal and post-natal clinics as well as carrying out deliveries. General practitioners were involved only with private patients, unless they had part-time contracts to cover local authority clinics or were prepared to respond to emergency calls from domiciliary midwives (Ferguson and Fitzgerald 1954: 29).

Despite the growth in both the supply of maternity beds and the demand from individual women for hospital confinements, official policy continued to assume the perpetuation of home deliveries. This view was supported by many women's organizations and by the medical profession. Even within the Royal College of Obstetricians and Gynaecologists which had been established in 1929 to institutionalize the development of the specialty, a majority expected the mix of hospital and domiciliary provision to continue into the indefinite future. For all the criticism of midwives and general practitioner obstetrics in the inter-war period, the remedy was seen to lie in improved training and incentives for better liaison rather than in abandoning their contribution to the process of childbirth. While home confinement might be predictable as official policy, given the lack of resources to invest in the scale of building that would have been needed to offer a hospital bed for every delivery, it is striking that no significant interest can be found arguing 'Hang the expense, hospital birth is the only safe policy, and the future health of the nation demands it and the money must be found'.

As so often in British social policy, it was the impact of war that brought lasting change, both in the effective national and local planning of health care services and in encouraging hospital deliveries. The government anticipated heavy bombing of civilian populations immediately upon the outbreak of hostilities and gave a high priority to the evacuation of pregnant women, mothers, and children from the expected target areas. This implied the provision of additional maternity services in the receiving areas. Accommodation was hastily commandeered and converted for use as maternity homes. Staff were redeployed to cover these. In practice, inevitably, the system did not work quite as expected. Women were reluctant to be moved or made their own alternative arrangements. The 'phoney war' over the winter of 1939/40 led many to drift home. As a result, maternity facilities were underutilized in the receiving areas. A new scheme was devised which simply moved women for their actual confinement, although the numbers involved were never large even when serious air raids began in September 1940.

But the destruction of housing and hospital accommodation and the difficulties of arranging domiciliary confinements in homes overcrowded by billeting eventually led to a crisis of provision. Women, in London particularly, were forced to use the emergency facilities in the countryside if a normal delivery was expected. Some of them beat the system by waiting for labour to start and then turning up at the local maternity hospital but most, albeit grudgingly, complied. The pressure was not relieved, however, because the birth rate continued to rise, reaching its highest levels since 1928 (Ferguson and Fitzgerald 1954: 27–52). The effect, though, was to give a substantial further boost to hospital confinements so that over half of all births were in hospital by 1945.

Maternity accommodation continued to be a problem throughout the war and into the early years of the NHS. During 1941, however, it was overtaken as a concern by the shortage of staff. Anxieties about this had been expressed, particularly by the voluntary hospitals, just before the war. The Ministry of Health and the CMB had taken the view that the dearth of pupils was a temporary phenomenon caused by a rush to train, before the course was lengthened in 1938, and a subsequent rebound. The creation of a full-time salaried service meant that former independent practitioners would be available for recruitment if the hospitals were willing to pay proper salaries rather than to rely on cheap pupil labour. By 1940, however, it was clear that the demand for midwifery training had not recovered and that wastage was increasing because of the attractions of other forms of war service. The ministry discussed a prohibition on midwives leaving their employment as early as 1941 but initially tried a combination of moral pressure with the work of the Rushcliffe Committee in reviewing salaries and conditions (p. 105).

This Committee reported in July 1943 (HMSO: 1943), but had already been overtaken by compulsory measures. The armed forces were barred from recruiting newly qualified and practising midwives; they were permitted to change jobs only through the Ministry of Labour. In September 1943, all midwives were compelled to remain in their present posts for six months, later extended by another three months, and newly qualified midwives had to practise for a year. This did not solve the problem of distribution, since the newly qualified often contrived to remain in their training hospitals so, in April 1944, the ministry used its powers to direct them to areas of shortage. Ironically, this achieved some effect in an unintended way. General nurses could avoid direction by entering midwifery training, boosting recruitment at the expense of tuberculosis, mental and chronic sick hospitals. Continuing shortages meant that these controls were maintained with some modification until June 1946 (Ferguson and Fitzgerald 1954: 284–331).

It is important to set the Rushcliffe Committee in this context because of the way it is often hailed by writers on midwifery as an historic assertion of their autonomy and status. Just as in the First World War, the diversion of doctors to military service made midwives more essential to both hospital and domiciliary services. They represented a form of dilution which allowed scarce medical resources to be concentrated on complicated deliveries. This, surely, is the significance of the finding from the RCOG/ Population Investigation Committee Survey *Maternity in Great Britain* (1948) that 75 per cent of deliveries in hospitals had been performed by midwives. The Rushcliffe Committee's work was conducted against a background of attempts by the Ministry of Health to keep midwives at work by persuasion, flattery and cajolery. When its report emphasized the independence of the midwife then, it may be more plausible to read this less as a reversal of the trend towards emphasizing her nursing background and auxiliary status than as part of the campaign to preserve the staffing of maternity services by voluntary means.

The continuing shortage of midwives persisted after the war and was seen as a potential constraint on the planning for a national health service. A major recruitment drive was launched at the end of 1945 but the slow response, partly because of the reluctance of employers to adopt the improvements in conditions advocated by the government, forced a further review and a Working Party on Midwives was set up in 1947. Its report (Ministry of Health 1949), in 1949, reiterated the Rushcliffe line, defining the midwife as the expert in normal childbearing with the doctor as her partner in dealing with the abnormal (Oakley 1984: 143–4).

In the meantime, however, the National Health Service had begun to destroy the economic basis of midwifery. They were no longer low-cost providers: all provision was free of charge at the point of service. Women now tended to make the general practitioner the first port of call to confirm a pregnancy and only to reach a midwife through him. While the NHS eliminated the previous economic competition between the GP and the midwife, it established her subordination. If a doctor and a midwife were present together at a delivery, NHS regulations gave him precedence and defined her as a maternity nurse (Oakley 1984: 143). It is a debatable question how far these developments should be seen as a deliberate attack on midwives, a response to the shortage or the chance oversight of busy planners. Given the evidence that the Ministry of Health was thinking of midwives as essentially maternity nurses in the 1920s, it is probably wrong to see this as more than a reversion to that tradition in the face of failure of measures to improve recruitment. Even if they had opted for a midwife-led service, it is not clear that sufficient midwives would have been available to provide it. Certainly the general practitioners did not benefit, since the rate of hospital confinements continued to rise throughout the 1950s. Indeed, general practice was in a state of some disorganization throughout this decade in the wake of staffing decisions by the regional review committees in 1948 which had creamed off some GPs into consultant appointments and expelled many more from any hospital work. The GPs were a residual category of second-class doctors with no clear identity, poor facilities and low morale. The repair of this condition was to be a major problem for the NHS in the 1960s (Stevens 1966: 96–105, 153–68, 286–319).

Although some GPs continued to retain an active interest in maternity services and were given incentives to do so, the real winners from the NHS were the hospital staff. From a planning viewpoint this is understandable, since it permitted more intensive use of scarce personnel and midwives remained in short supply throughout the 1950s and 1960s (Towler and Bramall 1986: 257). But the RCOG's rise from a private association, founded in 1929, to a Royal Charter, agreed in 1938 but not issued until 1946 (Stevens 1966: 45), came at exactly the right time for it to arrive in the councils of the medical establishment at the inception of the NHS. The regional review committees which played such a key role in subordinating general practice had a core membership of two physicians, two surgeons and one obstetrician/gynaecologist which was supplemented as necessary (Stevens 1966: 98). There was a generous supply of would-be specialists in training posts, which continued into the early years of the NHS, and the specialty managed to obtain a disproportionate share of distinction awards (Stevens 1966: 190–1, 281–9). The combined efforts of the ministry and the college had also established a relatively generous and well-distributed level of bed provision, when compared with areas like psychiatry or paediatrics.

The hospitals had been under stress during and immediately after the war as a result of the combination of enemy action and a high birth rate. Once the baby boom passed, however, after 1948, the NHS seems to have opted for a policy of keeping expensive beds occupied and letting the hospital confinement rate rise, rather than trying to close or redeploy these surplus resources. The inflexibility of the NHS capital stock is a long-standing problem: hospital space cannot change its use as freely and flexibly as retail space. By the time the Maternity Services Committee under Lord Cranbrook reported in 1959 (Ministry of Health, 1959), the birth rate had begun to rise again. But expectations had been created for both women and doctors about the availability of hospital beds, which were reflected in its report, suggesting provision for 70 per cent hospital confinements against the 1959 rate of 64.2 per cent. These estimates were incorporated into the building programmes of the 1960s which were the most significant capital investment since the NHS was established. However, by the time this capacity came on stream, the birth rate was declining again and the service faced the same problems of resource inflexibility. Again, the response was a rise in the hospital confinement rate to reach 98.6 per cent by 1980 (Macfarlane and Mugford 1984: 158).

This trend attracted relatively little resistance until the 1970s, although there were isolated critics from the early 1960s. Part of this reflects the intrinsic dynamic of modern medicine, namely that new technologies tend to appear first in hospitals and it is only with greater experience and development that they can be made sufficiently safe and portable for general use. In the early 1950s, domiciliary practitioners, whether doctors or midwives, still had less effective means of analgesia at their disposal than a hospital could offer (Towler and Bramall 1986: 241–2). By the end of that decade, the new methods of ultrasound investigation and active management with oxytocic drugs were becoming available in hospitals. Although these might have been confined to high-risk deliveries, research has had relatively little success at defining risk and establishing good predictors (Oakley 1984: 220–1). The problem is that no one can confidently define a labour as normal until it is complete and there is a well-established tendency in medicine to regard intervention as more professionally defensible than inaction in cases of uncertainty (Scheff 1963).

These external changes have had a considerable effect on midwifery. Their result has been to complete the transformation of the midwife into a maternity nurse. In describing the midwife as a 'maternity nurse', we do not mean to imply that her work has become any less skilled; indeed its technical content has increased substantially in the last twenty years. But this has turned the midwife into an extension of the doctor rather than an alternative practitioner. Since 1967, midwives have acquired the authority to administer perineal anaesthesia, perform and suture episiotomies, take blood from babies for various tests, intubate neonates, administer oxytocic drugs on their own initiative, manage and remove epidural catheters and administer intravenous infusions. Over the same period, the CMB had to abandon its requirement that pupil midwives should conduct a specified number of domiciliary deliveries and content itself with urging that pupils should receive instruction in natural as well as 'managed' labour. It is a process which is directly comparable to the long-term tendency in general nursing for the downward delegation of routinized, albeit skilled, medical tasks and techniques at the expense of the nurses' role as a spiritual or, in modern terms, psychological support for the patient.

Although the RCM maintains the fiction of the midwife as 'practitioner in her own right', this is not in any way comparable to the pre-war situation of the midwife as an independent practitioner. It amounts to little more than saying that the midwife must take responsibility for her own actions within a framework of rules defined by modern obstetric practice. There is a substantial zone of discretion, more than for many nurses, and the existence of a licensing board and its discipline represent a countervailing power to that of the midwife's employer. But the NHS midwife is not, for instance, personally liable to her patients in the event of an adverse outcome and possible litigation. The service she offers is set within a framework of policy and organization dictated by others and negotiable only within fairly narrow limits.

The extent of this change has been rather obscured by the impact of feminism upon midwifery and the formation of an alliance between midwives who are discontented with their subordinate role and women who want more control over their experience of childbirth. Their joint critique of contemporary obstetrics has had considerable media exposure and a high public profile. However, its practical effects are unclear. As Reid (1983: 84–91) has pointed out, discussing Oakley's work, the constituency of consumer support for radical change seems to be very limited. What her, mainly working-class, mothers wanted above all was a safe, clean, private and pain-free experience, all of which are more difficult to guarantee in the sort of housing that they had access to. They would certainly have preferred a more caring environment but that does seem to be what obstetricians have sought to provide in response to criticism. Most types of instrumental delivery, for example, have stabilized or declined since the late 1970s (DHSS 1986: Table 4.1). The movement has created a small private sector of like-minded mothers and midwives but, as Towler and Bramall (1986: 276) emphasize, this has a marginal and economically precarious existence.

Independent midwifery emerged under a very specific set of social and economic conditions which united the provision of a low-cost service to the poor with the desire of some middle-class women to establish female control over the process of childbirth. This alliance kept midwifery alive as an autonomous occupation while its economic and technological independence was steadily eroded. The absorption of the CMB by the UKCC structure after 1979 merely confirmed a *de facto* amalgamation which had been in process for half a century. The existence of a small private constituency may perpetuate some of the rhetoric of independence but it is hard to see that being re-established unless further social or economic change recreates the original conditions, by, for example, large-scale privatization of health care services and the deliberate stimulation of competition between providers to control costs. It is conceivable that midwives could come to be more important within the NHS as a cheaper alternative to doctors but this would not represent the kind of qualitative transformation demanded by the most vociferous advocates of professional autonomy but a consolidation of the nurses' traditional status as a skilled technician–assistant.

Chapter nine

District Nursing and Health Visiting

Midwifery is a technically specialized area of nursing work and, consequently, particularly vulnerable to the effects of developments in medical knowledge and technology. Its social relations, with clients and with the medical profession, are, however, very similar to those of other branches of nursing which emerged outside the hospitals. We have already discussed the work of handywomen and private duty nurses at some length, so that our account here begins directly from the official versions of the foundation of district nursing and health visiting. In discussing these, however, it is important to acknowledge the marked imbalance of primary scholarship on the two groups. This is not entirely coincidental: the importance of maternal and child welfare in national policy since the late nineteenth century (Gilbert 1966, Thane 1981, Titmuss 1958, Dwork 1986) has been accentuated by its interest to feminist social historians (e.g. Davin 1978, Dyehouse 1978, Lewis 1980) and to the debate between McKeown (1965) and his critics, especially Winter (1977, 1979, 1982), on the causes of improvements in infant mortality in the twentieth century. As a result, the policy context of developments in health visiting is relatively well defined and has been the subject of a number of specialized treatments (Davies 1988, Dingwall 1974, 1977b, 1983b, Robson 1983, 1986). District nursing, on the other hand, has been relatively neglected, apart from the useful books by Stocks (1960) and Baly (1987) on the history of the Queen's Institute. This partly reflects its very invisibility in policy debate. It was not a subject for repeated official investigations or government initiatives. Its past is not preserved in major official archives but in the scattered records of local voluntary associations which, if they have survived at all, are less readily located and more laborious to collate.

Nursing in the home
Histories of district nursing traditionally begin from the activities

173

of William Rathbone in Liverpool. (His involvement with the Poor Law Infirmary in that city was discussed in Chapter 4.) As a young man, Rathbone had been a voluntary visitor for the District Provident Society, distributing charitable relief in the poorest areas of the city. In 1859 he employed a woman called Mary Robinson, who had nursed his first wife through a terminal illness, to work among the sick poor. She was initially reluctant but both of them became persuaded of the value of her work and he decided to extend it. Rathbone made various attempts to interest existing bodies like St John's House or the Sisters of Charity. For a variety of reasons none of these organizations were able to assist and he turned to Florence Nightingale for advice. She gave him an interview and recommended that he should approach the Liverpool Royal Infirmary, a voluntary hospital, to accept women for training. A school was set up there in 1862. The probationers were shared between the hospital and the nursing association which the Rathbone family set up in 1861 to manage the scheme.

William Rathbone may well have been the first to use the term 'district nursing'. If we break down the elements of his scheme, however, it is possible to see that it was much less of an innovation than it is often made to appear.

As we showed in Chapter 2, and as Rathbone's own history illustrates, the idea of district visiting was not new. Associations for the provision of nursing care to the poor had been in existence for some twenty or thirty years under a variety of religious auspices. Similar organizations were still being founded: the Bible and Domestic Mission in London, for instance, began to provide visiting nurses from 1857 under the direction of Mrs Ranyard (Seymer 1954, Stocks 1960: 21–5, Baly 1987: 10). Although William himself was a Unitarian, the Rathbones were a Quaker dynasty within a tradition of social activism.[1] The division of labour between the ladies' committees which were set up to manage each district and the paid women is also a familiar one. Mary Robinson was actually an experienced nurse[2] from St Thomas's in the pre-Nightingale Fund era. The other staff were a mixture of women trained at the Infirmary or qualified 'by reason of long experience'. The appointments depended upon the resources and preferences of each district committee. As with the sisterhoods of the 1840s, these working-class women were closely supervised by a lady inspector in each district 'who goes round and enquires for herself into the general efficiency of the nurse' (Baly 1986: 125). Similar arrangements had been created where public funds were involved. The nurses hired by the Oxford Guardians in the 1854 cholera epidemic (p. 13) were monitored by a lady who visited every house to instruct the nurses to comfort the sick, to cheer the disconsolate and, where need was, herself to supply a sudden emergency, or to relieve a wearied attendant. (H.W. Ackland (1856) *Memoir of the Cholera Epidemic at Oxford in 1854*, Churchill, London. Quoted by Dean and Bolton 1980: 93)

A similar association was set up in Manchester in 1864 and recruited some nurses from King's College and St Thomas's for district work in 1867 (Bullough and Bullough 1979: 143, Baly 1987: 10). Its structure was adopted by the Manchester and Salford Ladies Sanitary Association. The 'mission woman' whom they employed in 1867 is often regarded as the first health visitor. The paid workers in Manchester and Salford were ordinary working-class women until 1907 when the local authority assumed responsibility for the service and decided to restrict future appointments to trained nurses (Simon 1938: 210). They lived in the poor districts where they worked, were paid a wage comparable to that of the people in the neighbourhood and received limited on-the-job training (Dingwall 1983b: 611–13). As one of the lady volunteers wrote in a paper read to the Ladies' Section of the Congress of the Royal Institute of Public Health at Blackpool, in 1899, 'the health visitor is usually a superior woman of the class sought to be helped . . . her home is naturally an object lesson in cleanliness, tidiness etc. to the neighbours who, of course, occupy exactly similar houses' (quoted by Davies 1988 cf. Smith 1979: 115). But these women were not trusted to work on their own. Each was partnered by a lady volunteer 'in charge of the district'. The ladies were involved partly in fund raising and partly in organizing meetings for working-class women in the district at which lectures on sanitary and health issues were given. Evidence given to the 1904 Inter-Departmental Committee on Physical Deterioration makes it clear that the recruitment of suitable lady supervisors was a more important constraint on the expansion of the scheme than the availability of 'sanitary mission women' (Dingwall 1983b: 611).

The form which these schemes took reflects two principles in the organization of mid-Victorian philanthropy which we have already identified. One is the co-option of working-class women to the task of maintaining order and social discipline. The other is the importance of the household as a model for the relationship between women from different social classes. The Ladies' Sanitary Reform Association in Manchester and Salford grew out of the limited success of a parallel male association formed in 1852. This body was one of a number of similar societies founded in the wake of the 1832 and 1848 cholera epidemics to lobby for permanent improvements in sanitary legislation and its enforcement rather than simply relying on transient responses to such crises, and to seek to educate working-class men by way of lecturing, leafleting and the display of posters in workplaces. The ladies' association in 1860 was set up because of the failure of these efforts. If men could not be persuaded directly to change their ways, perhaps they could be reached through their wives. But, again, simple exhortation seems to have been unsuccessful and the 'mission woman' became the means to reach right into the working-class home. The choice of terminology is significant. The term 'health visitor' did not come into use until about 1900 and the work was described in the language of urban evangelism. Dowling (1963) notes the influence of this model on the Ladies Sanitary Association and one of its leading theorists, Mrs Ranyard, had already advocated the use of a 'good poor woman' as a 'missing link' between Christian ladies and the classes in need of reform (Platt 1939: 62, 64). Her access, however, depended upon the provision of services which were not socially appropriate for lady volunteers; an element in early health visiting which is often overlooked. The 1867 'mission woman'

> had not only given instruction in common sanitary rules but she would herself wash and make comfortable a sick person whom she might find neglected or dirty, thus encouraging those who were around to follow her example by showing people how to do what was needful in the best way. (Langton 1963: 1248)

This was still the case in 1904 when health visitors in Manchester and Salford are described as 'making the beds of sick patients and cleaning their houses' (Dingwall 1983b: 612). As we saw in discussing nursing in the Crimea, manual labour of this kind was not considered acceptable for middle-class women. So both the Liverpool and the Manchester and Salford schemes perpetuated the mistress/servant relationship which had marked their predecessors in both hospital and home nursing services.

One other point which both schemes had in common was their willingness to provide financial relief as well as practical assistance (Baly 1986: 125–6, Dingwall 1983b: 612). This provoked an argument between William Rathbone and Florence Nightingale which is of great importance for the understanding of the latter's conception of home nursing.

Rathbone wrote to Florence Nightingale in 1874 on behalf of a group considering the formation of a District Nursing Association in London. Her initial response was hostile, pointing to the lack of evidence to establish the need but also attacking Rathbone's conception of its work. In Liverpool, she complained in a letter to Hilary Bonham Carter, 'the nurses did no dressings, no bed linen changing but they simply gave and the (patients) liked it' (quoted by Baly 1986: 126). This is a tendentious characterization of the Liverpool scheme which had done extensive work with TB and fever patients and made major contributions to the civic response to the cholera and typhoid epidemics of 1866 and 1870–1 (Stocks 1960: 31–7). But it does go to the heart of her objections.

To the extent that Florence Nightingale supported district nursing and health visiting, this reflected her basic hostility to hospital-based health care and the priority she gave to the reconstruction of Victorian society on sanitary principles. Home nursing was a means to that end, a way to separate the poor from each other rather than grouping them together in hospitals where they could be a mutually corrupting influence. *Notes on Nursing* (Nightingale 1859) emphasizes preventive work, 'nursing the well', encouraging resistance to disease and disseminating the moral laws of domestic hygiene. In this respect it is one of the first texts in the creation of what Armstrong (1983: 7–8) has called the Dispensary. This is a metaphor for the conceptual shift that extended medicine from the correction of the sick in specially segregated and regulated institutions to the social control of the healthy. The same vision permeates her writing, whether she is discussing sanitary missions to the poor of India or her brother-in-law's tenants in Buckinghamshire (Woodham-Smith 1950: 424). Home nursing, for her, was a civilizing occupation, reforming and redirecting the lives of its patients, not just caring for them.

This approach brought her close to the ideals of the Charity Organization Society.[3] The formation of the COS reflected a growing disillusion among philanthropists with the results of their labours. Neither exhortation nor personal examples of moral living and community service seemed to be yielding results in terms of changing working-class behaviour. There was an indiscriminate proliferation of charitable effort which led to waste and duplication and created opportunities for the undeserving and idle to manipulate the system in their favour. Gifts of relief, whether in cash, goods or services, destroyed the incentive to change. What was needed was a more rigorous and co-ordinated approach where those seeking assistance would have their background meticulously investigated, their needs scientifically measured and their compliance with prescriptions for social and economic behaviour carefully monitored. Those who were deemed responsible for their own misfortune or rejected the standards demanded of their future conduct would be denied private aid and forced onto the Poor Law. To fulfil its role as the ultimate means of social discipline, short of using criminal sanctions, it should be applied with a deterrent harshness (Stedman Jones 1971, Fido 1977, Garland 1985: 114–22).

Such a philosophy made quite different demands of its agents. In particular, they themselves must be people with a moral character inherently capable of withstanding the temptation to temper the exactitude of their approach out of sympathy with their clients and to withstand the interpersonal buffeting of investigative contacts with the poor. This implied a need to recruit from a higher social class and to give a more rigorous training, both of which are reflected in Florence Nightingale's approach to home nursing. She constantly underlines the differences between nursing inside hospital, where there is an elaborate system of discipline and control to structure the nurse's work, and nursing in the home where the nurse must rely on her personal qualities and skills.

> The District Nurse must . . . be of a yet higher class and of a yet fuller training than a hospital nurse . . . the doctor has no one but her to report to him. She is his staff of clinical clerks, dressers and nurses. (Quoted from F. Nightingale, *On Trained Nursing for the Sick Poor*, 1876 by Baly 1986: 128)

The list at the end of the quotation is revealing. The clerks and dressers were apprentice doctors, so that the boundary between medicine and nursing in the community appears to be rather different from that in the hospital. The hospital nurse is a subordinate craftsman, the 'building staff' to the medical 'architect' in one of her own metaphors. Her background is unimportant: what matters is training rather than origins or the receipt of payment (Cook 1913: 269–71). Her counterpart in the community is much closer to the doctor, as a treatment assistant.

The authentic expression of COS spirit can be found in her insistence that the district nurse and the sanitary missioner are not themselves agents of charity. In a letter to Lady Rosebery, Chairman of the Scottish Council of the Queen's Jubilee Institute, Florence Nightingale emphasized that

> Besides a nurse, she must be a sanitary missionary, for where doles are given, nursing flies out at the window or rather remains outside the door. But she must know what sanitary authorities to have recourse to, in what respects the necessary offices of a dwelling are deficient or neglected. She must also know to what charitable agencies to have recourse, when there

is a real want of food, clothing, bedding but especially of medical comforts. She is not herself to form another pauperising agency but to *depauperise*. (Original emphasis. Quoted by Ferguson 1958: 458)

This is underlined in her introduction to Rathbone's *History of District Nursing* (1890) where she observes that

Besides nursing the patient, she shows them in their own homes how they can call in official sanitary help to make their one poor room healthy, how they can improvise appliances, how their home need not be broken up. (Quoted by Baly 1986: 132)

Florence Nightingale's vision of the district nurse is that of a COS caseworker, a supervisor of the poor rather than a provider for them. In a sense, it could only be so: without the elaborate infra-structure of the hospital most nursing care in the home must always necessarily be provided by kin, friends or neighbours, unless the patient can afford and has space to board a private nurse. Here the relationship between mistress and servant is reproduced in a different form. The nurse is a repository of knowledge, both physical and social, which she can use to direct her patients to help themselves. She is not there to act for them but to make them act in accordance with her precepts. Indeed, by 1891, Florence Nightingale was even questioning the identification of this work with nursing, in her correspondence with Frederick Verney, Chairman of the North Buckinghamshire Technical Education Committee: 'it hardly seems necessary to contrast sick nursing with (health visiting) . . . (the health visitor) must create a new work and a new profession for women.' Cook (1913: 384) also records her as taking an interest in the expanding work of women sanitary inspectors in this field later in the 1890s.

The picture that emerges from these data, then, belies many of the simplifications imposed upon it in writing accounts of the development of nursing specialties. The home visiting schemes of Liverpool and of Manchester and Salford are not clearly distinguished in their organization, their personnel or their practice. Both grew out of existing traditions and were probably innovative only to the extent that they were less obviously sectarian than the sisterhoods of the 1840s. They shared the strategy of co-opting the handywoman class to perform its traditional role under a new system of control. But they cannot in any sense be said to be contributing to the formation of a self-conscious occupation. The ladies running the schemes may have had a serious purpose but they were essentially amateurs engaged in a subjective occupation.

The women whom they employed were recruited and trained on an ad hoc basis with job-specific skills. By the 1860s, there were serious criticisms of the adequacy of this model as a means of executing the civilizing mission of home nursing. If we are to identify the foundation of district nursing and health visiting as distinct occupations, we need to look elsewhere.

Drafting the middle classes

The modern shape of district nursing and health visiting owes most to two specific movements of organized social intervention; district nursing represents the professionalization of voluntary effort, in the sense that its successful execution was seen to turn on the use of trained specialists rather than well-informed amateurs; health visiting derives from the extension of municipal responsibilities for public health beyond sewers, drains and building structures.

William Rathbone's response to Florence Nightingale's criticism of his proposals for district nursing in London was to commission Florence Lees, one of the more able and experienced lady nurses from St Thomas's, to survey the existing provision. The report, published by the Metropolitan and National Association in 1875, showed that there were 26 societies in London, of which 11 supplied nurses with some sort of hospital-based training. There is little attempt to evaluate these schemes in detail, so much as to dismiss them in order to justify the assertion that a new association is needed founded on more systematic training than offered elsewhere, even at St Thomas's. The object must be to 'elevate nursing to the rank of a scientific art for educated women like that of the medical profession' (quoted by Baly 1986: 128). In this respect, Florence Lees's views anticipate those of the Bedford Fenwick faction in the struggle over registration (cf. Stocks 1960: 44, Baly 1987: 12–16). Her emphasis on the recruitment of lady probationers and a high level of technical education was a cause of some friction with Miss Nightingale's associates and, occasionally, Miss Nightingale herself. However, Florence Nightingale's own views on district nursing seem to have muted her opposition to Miss Lees. While she did not want to close the door on 'common women', she accepted that the district nurse would require a higher standard of character and skills which could have the effect of excluding working-class candidates.

The Metropolitan and National Association for Providing Trained Nurses for the Sick Poor was established in 1875 with Florence Lees as its first superintendent. It was partly financed by the Nightingale Fund until 1881 and Henry Bonham Carter, the fund's secretary, was a member of its committee for many years. The Duke of Westminster was the first chairman. This connection was important because he was also appointed one of the trustees of the Women's Jubilee Offering in 1887. This was a fund subscribed by the women of Britain to mark the fiftieth anniversary of Queen Victoria's accession to the throne. After considerable intrigue the Queen was persuaded to allocate the bulk of it to support the nursing of the sick poor in their own homes. Although, as Stocks (1960: 63–72), Smith (1982: 168) and Baly (1987: 18–25) note, there was some disagreement over the exact disposition of the funds, the Metropolitan Association was clearly endorsed as the model, not least by Florence Nightingale in her advice to another trustee, Sir James Paget (Cook 1913: 355).

The result was the foundation of the Queen Victoria Jubilee Institute for Nursing the Poor in their Own Homes in 1889. Although 15 local societies employing 91 nurses had affiliated by the end of 1890, the Metropolitan Association dominated and was adopted as the national centre for training. The first Inspector-General was William Rathbone's niece, Rosalind Paget, who was a leading member of the Midwives Institute. Most of her experience was hospital based – she had trained as a nurse at the London – and it is revealing that she elected to work with the Metropolitan Association in 1889 to gain experience for organizing the Institute (Cowell and Wainwright 1981: 22). She held the appointment only until September 1891 but she then joined the council of the institute and remained an important link between the developments in district nursing and midwifery. She was later the Institute's first nominee on the Central Midwives Board, for example.

From the start the institute tried to impose a high entrance requirement on its probationers and insisted that its affiliates should employ only fully trained women as nurses. The result was that relatively few nurses were trained by the institute – only 539 by 1896 – and a good proportion of the district nursing around the country continued to be provided by associations of ladies employing ordinary women on the Liverpool model (Baly 1986: 134–5). The Queen's Nurses seem to have been similar in background to the hospital nurses of this later period. Stocks (1960: 89) refers to four daughters of clergymen, one stockbroker, two 'merchants', an Oxford professor, a music teacher, a solicitor, a bank manager, a works manager, a commercial traveller, an auctioneer, an engineer, a farmer and a Major-General. In fact, as Donnison (1977: 141–2) points out, the Queen's Nurses were reluctant to work in rural areas since neither the salaries on offer nor the fees that could be generated were adequate compensation for the social deprivations and the hostility of local medical practitioners, who felt threatened by these 'new professionals'. By 1896, the institute was forced to compromise its principles and start training 'Village Nurses', ordinary women who would return to their own homes and act as nurse–midwives in the locality (Baly 1987: 54–55). The difficulties of providing care in rural areas if recruitment standards were set too high exemplified the crucial policy dilemma which the midwives had also faced, between trying to exclude the handywoman or trying to incorporate her in a more disciplined and regulated structure.

The institute's emphasis on high standards of training and a subordinate role for lay committees weakened its influence nationally. As Stocks (1960: 95, 136–7, 124–30) shows, district nursing associations in major cities like Bristol and Newcastle-upon-Tyne refused to affiliate and there was open conflict between Liverpool, which affiliated in 1898, and London during 1907–9 over the latter's attempt to impose a syllabus and examinations that disadvantaged the less-educated women who were being recruited on Merseyside. The issue of village nurses was also a divisive one. Although the institute had been forced to give them some limited recognition, their attempt to impose a rigid administrative separation between the two classes of nurse was seen in areas like Hampshire as an obstruction to economical and effective management and to the gradual substitution of Queen's Nurses for village nurses as trained staff and funds permitted. Northumberland disaffiliated in 1901 because of its differences with national institute policy on this issue. The Ranyard Mission remained outside in order to retain its denominational character. Indeed, the institute's insistence on the non-sectarian character of its work caused a number of conflicts especially, but not exclusively, in Ireland. There was also a significant competition from the Cottage Benefit Nursing Association set up in 1883 by Mrs Broadwood. By 1909 this had 131 affiliates and about 40 other groups associated with its principles, employing, in total, about 800 women. They received a few months' simple training in London and worked as living-in nurses with the poor, who paid by subscribing to a provident fund. They were much more popular with the doctors (Stocks 1960: 133–4, Baly 1987: 56).

District nursing remained dominated by voluntary associations until the 1950s. Before reviewing its later development and nationalization, though, it may be more useful to examine the alternative path represented by the emergence of health visiting. Unlike district nursing, it has no very clear antecedents in the care of the sick at all. It derives, rather, from the attempt to take over and order other aspects of the handywoman's work, particularly as a fixer of the problems of unwanted children and as an adviser on the care of those who were retained.

Concern about 'baby-farming', the placing of unwanted infants for adoption, had been growing in medical circles since the early 1860s. After some controversy, parliament passed an Infant Life Preservation Act in 1872 which required anyone caring for two or more children under one year of age for more than one day for payment to register with the relevant local authority. The act itself was largely ineffective (Behlmer 1982: 38–40, Rose 1986: 162). Nevertheless, a few authorities, especially the Metropolitan Board of Works and its successor, the London County Council, made serious efforts at enforcement and appointed inspectors to carry out the work.

Although in purely numerical terms the Infant Life Preservation inspectors are marginal to the history of health visiting, the legislation itself was of considerably more significance in three ways. First, it introduced a new principle in an inspection of private homes which went beyond the established power to examine and remedy structural defects in sanitation which threatened the public health. It accepted that child care might be a private affair but it was one that had public implications (Dingwall and Eekelaar 1988). Second, its very ineffectiveness guaranteed an active lobby to demonstrate its inadequacies and campaign for reforms. Paradoxically, it kept child welfare on the political agenda where a more rigorous statute might have killed it as an issue. Third, such attempts at enforcement as were made provided important evidence about the actual conditions under which children were living. The LCC inspectors followed up advertisements and maintained close liaison with police, relieving officers and registrars of births and deaths. But they also developed an advisory role on infant care and sanitation which represented a voluntary extension of their statutory duties (Behlmer 1982: 155).

The other important factor in the situation was the declining birth rate. As Dingwall (1977b) has shown, this was a major concern for the Interdepartmental Committee on Physical Deterioration whose report in 1904 gave the critical impetus to the state sponsorship of health visiting. If fewer children were being born, there was a national interest in maximizing the physical and moral quality of those who would become citizens. But this was not a new concern in 1904, although it had been crystallized by the debate of the Boer War. Alongside the humanitarian outrage of those Christian activists who saw cruelty to children as a symptom of the moral degeneracy of their times, we can trace a growing organizational concern with the future of the country as a commercial and military power (Dingwall *et al.* 1984).

The urgency of this problem for a great Imperial nation was partly responsible for the reappraisal of the pure COS programme during the 1880s and 1890s. The rigours of scientific casework, backed by the coercion of starvation or the Poor Law, were softened by the development of what Canon Barnett, one of its leading theorists, was to call 'practicable socialism'. It continued to emphasize the importance of individual character and personal morality but proposed that respectability should be rewarded by positive entitlements to state assistance in time of need (Garland 1985: 120–2). In alliance with the interventionist philosophies of public health medicine, the idea that even one 'missed case' was a public danger which must be sought out and treated, practicable socialism began to reconstruct the role of local government. In particular, it contributed to the rise of what Donzelot (1980: 82–95) discusses as the 'tutelary relationship' between families and the state. The surveillance of families could be extended by transforming its nature. Instead of the rigorous investigation of the caseworker, home visits would be occasions for the respectable poor to display their respectability and to be rewarded for it. Conversely, to deny entry would be a token of their disreputability and a legitimate cause for corrective interventions (Dingwall *et al.* 1984).

This process can easily be made to sound coherent and logical with hindsight. In practice, of course, it proceeded in a highly piecemeal fashion with a great deal of conflict and uncertainty about the outcome. The same period was marked not merely by competition with the COS advocacy of social policing but also with eugenic ideas which incited the abandonment of the poorest and weakest members of the society. Both the Poor Law and private charity, it was argued, merely encouraged the reproduction of the socially unfit to the exclusion of the better examples of the British race (Gilbert 1966, Garland 1985: 112–58).

One of the features of practicable socialism was its renewed emphasis on the virtues of personal contact between members of different classes, reflected best perhaps in the foundation of urban settlements such as Toynbee Hall where privileged young men could live and act among working-class communities. Although the municipal pioneers of home visiting did not go quite that far, the same thinking seems to have dominated. As Davies (1988) stresses, the exact pattern of the Manchester scheme was not repeated elsewhere. Instead, the emphasis returned to the use of middle-class women, either as employees of the Medical Officer of Health or as members of voluntary associations under his direction. Where the District Auditor was accommodating as in Worcestershire (1898) or Birmingham (1899), these appointments were of 'lady health missioners', 'women visitors', or 'lady health visitors' in spite of the absence of any clear statutory authority for such posts. Elsewhere, however, they were nominally employed as sanitary inspectors. The earliest appointments seem to have been in Glasgow in 1870 but the main initiative followed the passage of the Factories and Workshops Act 1891. By 1904, there were women sanitary inspectors in Preston, Longton, Burslem, Sheffield, Nottingham, Kensington, Leeds, Bradford and St Helen's (Dingwall 1977b, Davies 1988, Dwork 1986).

It was this model of middle-class employment which was endorsed by the 1904 Interdepartmental Committee in its call for the national provision of a 'health visiting' service (Dingwall 1983b: 616). In effect, it parallels the reform of midwifery envisaged by the Midwives Act 1902. Unlike midwifery, however, there was no clear lead given in identifying relevant qualifications or setting up licensing provisions.

Despite the lack of central initiative from the Local Government Board, there was a good deal of local response to the committee's proposals. An effective post-natal visiting service was made possible when the Notification of Births Act 1907 gave local authorities the power to require anybody attending the delivery of a baby to notify the Medical Officer of Health within thirty-six hours.[4] Previously information was not available until a birth was registered, which might take up to six weeks. The act did not specifically authorize authorities to employ health visitors and, indeed, the authorities were only compelled to operate it when further legislation followed in 1915. Manchester, for example, did not introduce notification of births until 1912. On the other hand local authorities could get LGB permission to implement the 1907 Act only if they undertook to set up a home visiting scheme (Lane-Claypon 1920: 10). This involved them in the identification of suitably educated staff, either to carry out the visits or to direct volunteer visitors. The power of the theory of separate spheres, the idea held by many feminists, as well as by men, that women had distinctive skills in dealing with questions of nurturance, ensured that these staff would have to be women. The authorities also had to find legal means of engaging staff without councillors being liable to surcharge for exceeding their powers.

Some authorities, like Huddersfield, where compulsory birth notification was pioneered under a local act of 1906, used women doctors, appointed as Assistant MOHs, to direct volunteer lady workers (Parton 1981). The use of volunteers in home visiting continued in some areas for a long time. Edinburgh employed one health visitor in 1914 to supervise 300 volunteers (Ferguson 1958: 544) and Oxford leant heavily on them until the early 1930s (Peretz, in press).

But there were few women doctors to form the core of a national service and reliable volunteers were hard to find. The recruitment of ladies in Manchester and Salford had always been troubled by their irregular commitment and the problems of imposing a uniform approach on people not subject to any formal work discipline (Dingwall 1983b: 610–13, cf. Lane-Claypon 1920: 110–1). Most areas, then, looked to modifications in the work of their women sanitary inspectors. This proved a highly contentious development.

Women sanitary inspectors had originally been recruited on a basis of equality with men, receiving the same salary, working under the same conditions and studying for the same qualifications. Although, in practice, they specialized in dealing with women workers and domestic hygiene, they were also competent to inspect cattle markets, slaughterhouses, sewage disposal and similar offensive environments. While this policy had important defenders, like Dr Cameron, the MOH for Leeds, it aroused considerable repugnance in other quarters. Many men and women were disturbed by the exposure of women inspectors to such experiences. Could they continue to cherish the finer qualities of their sex when their 'petticoats trailed in blood'? The male inspectors, in particular, saw this argument as a way of eliminating potential competitors in an overcrowded market for employment. While the women inspectors recognized the force of the claim that they had a unique potential for work on feminine matters, they also understood that once their work was separated from that of the men, its status would rapidly decline. The health visitor was seen as a dilution of sanitary inspection with a more limited training and a narrower range of work (Davies 1988, Dwork 1986: 126–9).

Ultimately the women sanitary inspectors were to lose. The Royal Sanitary Institute introduced a health visitor's certificate as a lower-level alternative to a sanitary qualification in 1908. This received legal recognition in 1909 in an order under the London County Council (General Powers) Act 1908. It was this act that first gave any local authority the power to appoint health visitors as such. The list of recognized qualifications suggests a strong emphasis on medical or nursing backgrounds. The boroughs could recruit women with either (a) a medical degree; (b) full nurse training; (c) the Certificate of the Central Midwives Board; (d) some nurse training and the Health Visitor's Certificate of an organization approved by the Local Government Board; or (e) previous experience with a local authority. Women sanitary inspectors would have qualified only under the last clause unless they chanced to have one of the other qualifications.

The Women Sanitary Inspectors' Association responded in two ways. First, it attempted to defend its sanitary inspector members by admitting health visitors and campaigning for better regulation of their pay and conditions so that they did not represent a cheaper and less-skilled alternative. Second, it successfully lobbied against a similar bill proposed by the Local Government Board in 1910 which would have explicitly authorized local authorities outside London to appoint health visitors but allowed each area freedom to decide what qualifications they should have. Despite the legal uncertainties, however, local authorities pressed ahead, circumventing the WSIA opposition by extending the duties of other authorized posts such as midwifery supervisors appointed under the 1902 Act or school nurses appointed under the Education (Administrative Provisions) Act 1907 which required medical inspection to be provided for children in elementary schools. This latter mode of development has been described in some detail for Durham (Dwork 1986: 202–4, Robson 1986). New appointments of women as sanitary inspectors dried up and, as existing staff left, duties were reallocated and posts regraded at a lower level. The title of health visitor came into general use for this new range of jobs.

Apart from the aesthetic objections to women sanitary inspectors, their cause was not helped by the way in which health visiting was explicitly contrasted with sanitary inspection as a mode of state action. Dr Bostock Hill, the MOH for Warwickshire and a leading advocate of health visiting, summed this up in a passage quoted with approval by Sir George Newman, later Chief Medical Officer to the Ministry of Health.

She is not an inspector in any sense of the word. Her functions are rather those of a friend of the household to which she gains access, and it is very gratifying to know that although at first there may have been some opposition to her entering a house, this rapidly died away, and in numerous instances she has been asked to return and aid the mothers of families by her help and counsel. In this new departure of carrying sanitation into the home, I believe we have not only an important but almost the only means of improving the health of the people. Sanitary authorities by providing water supply, drainage and decent houses have done much. In the future, however, the most important advice will come from an appreciation by the people themselves of the value of good health. (Newman 1906: 263–4)

Davies (1988) underlines the prevalence of this image of the health visitor as the mother's friend in the contemporary literature. It is, however, this that makes the relationship characteristic of tutelage, that social control is exercised invisibly through the desire to maintain a relationship with a representative of authority that confers approval and advertises respectability.

This analysis helps to make sense of the reports of client reactions. Bostock Hill acknowledges the opposition that these visits could arouse and it is not difficult to find negative reports (Smith 1979: 117, Lewis 1980: 106–7). Roberts (1973: 77–80), however, gives a much more positive reaction in his account of a slum childhood in Salford at the turn of the century and it is clear that the provision of health visiting rapidly became a political demand of organizations representing working-class women. The first woman sanitary inspector in Aberdeen was appointed in 1903 as a result of representations from the Union of Women (Dingwall 1974: 124) and both Lewis (1980) and Dwork (1986: 216–9) give additional evidence of support from groups like the Women's Co-operative Guild and the Women's Labour League. The point is that the support appears to have come from precisely that stratum of the respectable working class which practicable socialism aimed to recruit and co-opt to the maintenance of moral order and which has also traditionally provided the base of the British Labour movement (Pelling 1968). The bifurcation of working-class reactions to health visiting marks the success of the tutelary strategy. Middle-class women remained largely unexposed to health visiting until the 1920s. Health visiting was thus a more class-bound service than many subsequent accounts have suggested.

Nevertheless, there is nothing here that specifically identifies health visiting as having a natural kinship to general nursing in the way that district nursing and midwifery were identified as specialist skills to be based on an initial hospital training. A number of the early women sanitary inspectors and health missioners happened to be nurses but it is clear that this was a background that was regarded as useful rather than essential.

The process by which health visiting was captured as a branch of nursing is not well understood. However, two elements certainly need to be considered. One is the nature of the demand. These jobs were located in public health departments controlled by doctors who would, by this date, have been exposed to the use of women with some education as nurses in general hospitals. Nurses were a kind of auxiliary with which they were familiar. Moreover, some of the posts on which health visiting was based had an identifiable clinical component. School nurses, for example, performed a considerable number of minor treatments in clinics (Dwork 1986: 204–5).

On the supply side, it must be observed that, with the possible exception of certified teachers, it is not clear where else large numbers of women with a level of education intermediate between a board school and a degree could be found. More needs to be known about the market for different kinds of female labour at this period. Certainly, in a personal communication (1982), Davies has suggested that the market for trained nurses was slackening from the mid-1890s as opportunities for private duty work contracted and hospitals substituted cheaper, student labour. Some support for this thesis is provided by Baly (1986: 211) who notes that, in 1914, only 18 out of 45 St Thomas's nurses found hospital employment on completing their training. From about 1909, the nursing press was regularly carrying articles extolling health visiting as a career for ambitious nurses. The pay may have been lower than that of a sanitary inspector but it was still high by nursing standards and, as local government staff, health visitors undeniably enjoyed better arrangements for pensions and leave and more carefully regulated hours of work.

Even so, the work remained open to non-nurses well into the 1920s. Some restriction came with the LGB's recommendation in 1916 that local authorities should only appoint women as health visitors if they had two qualifications from: a recognized nurse training, the Certificate of the Central Midwives Board, or a Certificate from the Royal Sanitary Institute. Since most certified midwives with enough education to be eligible for health visitor posts would probably have had a general nurse training, this was likely to have been more restrictive than it appears. However, the LGB's central grants to support health visiting staff from 1918 went back to the 1909 LCC Order in their definition of qualified employees and when the Board of Education issued its first regulations on health visitor training in 1919, it offered two routes to qualification, neither of which particularly favoured nurses.

We are running somewhat ahead of ourselves here and we shall return to the question of the incorporation of health visiting by nursing at a later point in this chapter. If we pause, however, on the eve of the First World War, we can sum up the contrasts between district nursing and health visiting. District nursing was probably the larger in 1914: there were 2,096 Queen's Nurses at work, to say nothing of trained nurses employed by unaffiliated organizations and the semi-skilled village or cottage nurses (Stocks 1960: 147). In the same year, local authorities were employing 600 health visitors (Dwork 1986: 211). By this date, it is likely that this figure covers all public employees performing health visiting duties but, again, there is a penumbra of volunteers and staff employed by voluntary organizations but linked to local authorities whose exact size is unknown.

Unlike health visiting, however, district nursing had not been accepted as a proper object of public provision. In 1909, only about 3.5 per cent of the costs of Queen's Nurses and 1.6 per cent of the costs of village nurses associated with the institute came from public funds (Stocks 1960: 142). The histories of the Queen's Institute return repeatedly to its financial insecurity. Little change seems to have occurred by 1914, although there was some benefit from the National Insurance Act 1911 which led to agreements between approved societies and nursing associations to pay for home nursing care. In so far as there were any medical links at all, they were with general practitioners, many of whom were suspicious if not hostile to people whom they perceived as potential competitors. Health visiting, on the other hand, was fully accepted as part of the state health services. Even where voluntary workers were still involved, their activities were supervised, directed and often largely financed by local authorities. Health visitors were a vital extension of the Medical Officers of Health in their surveillance of local populations. District nursing, like midwifery, still had an uncertain margin between the trained practitioner and the handywoman. Health visiting, however, was firmly established as an organized occupation for educated women with its own representative association contrasting with the oligarchic structure of the Queen's Institute and its lay-dominated council.

These differences continued to shape the two areas of work through two world wars and into the National Health Service. District nursing remained marginal to the state, although increasingly.identified as a branch of nursing. Health visiting became increasingly important as the state became involved in problems of maternity and child welfare but remained marginal to nursing.

Home nursing and the state

As Titmuss (1958: 75–87) has observed, many of the key

developments in English social policy have been driven by the experience of war. Maternity and child welfare services in general were the beneficiaries of the First World War. By 1918, the number of health visitors employed by local authorities had more than quadrupled to 2,577 (Dwork 1986: 211). In contrast, the number of Queen's Nurses actually declined slightly to 1,999 (Stocks 1960: 147). Although there were few innovations in the form of service provision during the war, there was a steady programme of public investment. This was partly related to the perceived need to conserve infant lives to make good the losses of the war (Dingwall 1977b: 302–3, Robson 1986: 34–5, Dwork 1986: 208–20) although, as Gilbert (1970: 102–3) shows, it was facilitated by the rivalry between the chief medical officers at the Board of Education and the Local Government Board. These developments were checked by the hostility of the health insurance industry but were ultimately consolidated under the Maternity and Child Welfare Act 1918, which required local authorities to set up special committees with at least two women members and extended their power to make grants for a variety of institutional and domiciliary facilities. The LGB increased its recommended health visitor/population ratio from its 1915 estimate of 1 per 500 births to 1 per 400 and restricted its support for salaries to women qualified under the 1909 Order for London. It accepted the practice of using district nurse/midwives as health visitors in rural areas and recommended that health visitors should take over responsibility for infant life protection from boards of guardians by local arrangement. The LGB also advised that volunteers should be used only under the supervision of trained and paid staff and their most useful function was in assisting at clinics rather than in home visiting.

The increased resources available for health visiting during and after the war led to a number of qualitative changes in the work of health visitors. Perhaps the most important of these was the strengthening of control by the medical officer of health, especially in urban areas. Although voluntary agencies continued to be significant in the provision of clinical facilities, running 675 out of 1583 infant welfare centres in 1919 (Lane-Claypon 1920: 81), they were so dependent on local government funding as to have lost any real autonomy. Their role in home visiting, even simply following-up selected cases after an initial assessment by a health visitor, was in terminal decline. The only partial exception was the part played by County Nursing Associations in rural areas which we shall examine shortly.

The increased number of health visitors made it possible to

consider enlarging the scope of their work and giving them additional statutory duties. The exact pattern of their work seems to have varied considerably. Some areas developed forwards from the visiting of new babies throughout the pre-school period to link with the school medical services. Others worked backwards from their services to schools. In some areas health visitors took on work under tuberculosis, venereal disease and mental health legislation. Where it was difficult to persuade local GPs to accept certain duties, like the investigation of stillbirths, health visitors might be given the work, simply in order to get it done at all. A particular development was their involvement in ante-natal care. This was seen as a threat by some GPs, although others welcomed the extra referrals from the health visitors' monitoring. It aroused particular hostility from midwifery leaders, who were jealous of their own autonomy, but was an important back-up for the untrained midwives who remained significant service providers in poor communities. In such cases, health visitors would also take over responsibility earlier in the post-natal period, after 2–3 rather than 10–14 days (Lane-Claypon 1920).

Health visitors also became more involved with middle-class families. This was still a question which was treated with some delicacy and the actual policy was left to local decision. Nevertheless, writers like Janet Lane-Claypon, a medical officer with the LGB and the Ministry of Health and later Dean of the Household and Social Services Department at King's College for Women, were regarding this as good practice by 1920. Even well-to-do families merited a quarterly visit (Lane-Claypon 1920: 16–17, 31–2). It is not clear to what extent this aspiration was ever actually implemented: suburban middle-class districts in Manchester, for instance, were not covered by health visitors until 1929 (HMSO 1937: 91) and it seems doubtful whether there was enough health visitor time available to achieve this target for any class. Nevertheless, it was part of a transformation which made motherhood among the middle classes as much of a 'problem' as it was among the working class. The continued decline in the birth rate raised questions about the need for all women to be educated about their responsibilities for the future of the nation (Lewis 1980: 13–21).

Lane-Claypon (1920: 91–100) also underlines the difficulties of work in rural areas. Her analysis of the problem faced by service providers in the days before mass ownership of motor cars or telephones is worth quoting:

It is difficult for those who are not well acquainted with the conditions of rural England and Wales to realise the time taken to get about some of the areas. The train services on the small local lines are usually infrequent and inconvenient. The main roads are usually good but the by roads are often very bad in the winter. Some of the remoter houses have no road near them, and are a mile or more away from other houses. . . . Bicycling is almost essential for a visitor in a rural area. . . . The area which can be served . . . is about 2–2½ miles in radius. (Lane-Claypon 1920: 92, 95)

Outside the market towns, even the combination of infant welfare, school health, and tuberculosis control visiting would rarely generate enough work in a sufficiently compact area to justify a full-time employee.

In many rural areas, the solution was for the county council to contract with the County Nursing Association for a part of the time of district nurse/midwives to be given over to health visiting. While this did ensure that rural communities received some sort of service, it was never regarded as a wholly satisfactory arrangement. The existence of a County Nursing Association was no guarantee that the whole county was actually covered and a number of district associations preferred not to affiliate in order to preserve their autonomy. Most of their employees were village nurse–midwives with only twelve months' training divided between district nursing and midwifery. Although they might have reasonable practical skills they were not trained in child health work and were often unable to keep adequate records. Administrative responsibility was divided between the MOH and the nursing superintendent of the County Association, who was more likely to be a Queen's Nurse. Their policies and objectives might well be in competition if not necessarily in conflict. Finally the public health side of the work was always vulnerable to neglect because the nurse–midwives' work was more responsive to clinical demands.

As a matter of local policies, however, such contractual arrangements had their attractions as a device for providing some public subsidy to the county nursing associations. With the exception of payments for the nursing of specified diseases, there was no other statutory authority for local authorities to subsidize district nursing. Although they could give grants to sustain midwifery, these might be disproportionate to the volume of work in very isolated areas. The nursing associations were experiencing severe financial difficulties as a consequence of war-time inflation and were unable to rebuild their funds in the depressed economy of the inter-war years. Even the Queen's Institute was in trouble during the early part of the period. The injection of local authority funds contributed to the survival of district nursing/midwifery even if it only brought nearer the day when it would also be absorbed by the state health services (Lane-Claypon 1920: 91–100, Stocks 1960: 145–51).

In the early 1920s, the link between health visiting and nursing was still far from clearly forged. Lane-Claypon (1920: 145–51) presents the matter as one which reflected the personal preference of the local MOH. Nurses trained in hospitals knew little of normal health and domestic hygiene but they had acquired good habits of order and discipline. Midwifery training, particularly if it included some district experience, was more relevant but still covered only a small part of the work. Certainly, the Ministry of Health seems to have had an open mind on the question when it advised the Board of Education on the regulations for health visitor training issued in 1919. Lane-Claypon (1920: 105) hints that part of the motive for these may actually have been to draw intending health visitors away from midwifery training since there was concern about the limited number of certified midwives going into practice and the dearth of institutional deliveries made it difficult to increase training places.

Two routes to certification were prescribed for health visitors: a two-year course for candidates without previous training or experience and a one-year course for trained nurses, graduates, and women with three years' experience as health visitors (Ministry of Health 1919).

The regulations envisaged theoretical and practical instruction in elementary physiology, 'artisan cookery', general hygiene with particular reference to infants and children, the care of infectious diseases and minor ailments in children, an introduction to maternity work and an outline of the methods and objects of social work. Hutt's (1921: 372) textbook intended for this course suggests that the two-year training with entry at 18 was expected to be the normal route to qualification. By 1923, twenty-nine centres were offering training (McCleary 1935: 35) and the ministry issued a regulation in 1924 prohibiting the appointment of uncertificated health visitors by local authorities after 1 April 1928. This did not, however, affect staff employed by voluntary agencies so that the county nursing associations were not required to change their practice.

At some point in this period, however, candidates from a nursing background seem to have become dominant. The reasons for this remain obscure. There has been speculation that women from the two-year training lacked maturity (McEwan 1957: 24) although this is not represented as a problem in midwifery which permitted direct entry to a shorter training at a similar age. It may simply have been an unplanned development reflecting the changing demands of the work and the economic circumstances of local authorities. Clearly, some aspects, especially tuberculosis and school medical inspections, benefitted from a nursing background, although entrants via the two-year course were also required to undertake six months' hospital experience. In 1925, the ministry also seems to have changed its mind on the desirability of a previous midwifery training and made it a requirement for all new entrants. Again, the reasons for this change have not been explored. It seems curiously at odds with their efforts to keep the two occupations distinct by, for instance, discouraging the appointment of health visitors as inspectors of midwives and emphasizing the extent to which both ante- and post-natal care should really be given by midwives where trained practitioners were available (Lane-Claypon 1920: 132–3, Ministry of Health 1919). This requirement may reflect the extent to which health visitors were, in reality, still covering untrained or handywoman midwives.

Midwifery training had been extended in 1924 to six months for trained nurses and twelve months for direct entrants. The post-nursing health visitor course was cut to six months to accommodate this requirement but it had the effect of extending the training of other students by a year. Whereas a nurse would only have to find support, from her own resources or from a local authority, for six months, others would have to finance up to two years' education. Presumably, the pool of women qualified by experience for the one-year course was contracting and it is not clear that the salaries offered were particularly attractive to graduates. One possibility, given the evidence of continuing concern about the quality of independent midwifery in the late 1930s (HMSO 1937: 252), is that the employment of midwife-trained health visitors was seen as a way of providing some support and advice to mothers without the conflict and expense which would be provoked by direct public provision. But it may be more important to emphasize simple financial considerations in the deteriorating economic climate of the late 1920s. The number of training centres fell to 15 in 1933 and the number of full-time equivalent health visitors reached only 2,592 in that year, which represents virtually no increase on 1918 (McCleary 1935: 35–6). By 1938, there were 2,598 full-time equivalent health visitors employed by local authorities and a further 472 equivalents working for voluntary associations contracting to provide maternity and child welfare services (Ferguson and Fitzgerald 1954: 146). This did, in fact, represent a substantial improvement in the health visitor/population ratio largely because of the falling birth rate, in line with the ministry's 1934 target of 1 health visitor per 250 births. Nevertheless, it also suggests that new investment in maternity and child welfare services was actually going elsewhere.

At the outbreak of the Second World War, one of the most serious problems in the maternity and child welfare provision was seen to be the fragmentation between different types of hospital, local authority, and general practitioner services (Ferguson and Fitzgerald 1954: 29). The situation was compounded in district nursing by the proliferation of local associations and the jealousy with which they struggled to preserve their autonomy. We have already mentioned the financial difficulties of this sector and the tension between seeking local government subsidy and losing independence of action. The Queen's Institute tried to tackle this problem by promoting the development of local provident funds but these created their own problems, especially in the development of a lay, male bureaucracy to collect and administer them.

When local authorities took over the administration of the Poor Law in 1929, they also assumed responsibility for funding voluntary agencies. The money now came in the form of a block grant to the local authority rather than directly from the ministry or as an earmarked grant which the authority had to pass on. Local authorities, then, might prefer to use the funds to support their own staff rather than incurring the costs of administration involved in making grants to district nursing associations. In some areas, this was compounded by the antagonism between the patrician philanthropists who ran the nursing associations and the Queen's Institute and local authorities particularly, but not exclusively, those under Labour control who wanted to provide a co-ordinated nursing service as an entitlement rather than as an act of charity. When the London County Council took over responsibility for the Poor Law in 1929, for instance, the Queen's Institute was acknowledged for the quality of its work and numerical dominance but firmly sidelined as a force in policy making (Stocks 1960: 145–58, 173–5).

The institute's writ ran more strongly elsewhere. As might be expected, its leaders were enthusiastic supporters of registration and urged all Queen's Nurses to register. At the outbreak of the war there were 4,566 of them employed in Great Britain and Ireland (Stocks 1960: 159, 168). However, it is clear from other passages in Stocks's account that this is unlikely to represent the total district nursing workforce. In 1953, for example, local authorities had come to employ 9,203 district nurses of whom only

4,032 were Queen's Nurses (Stocks 1960: 196). It seems unrealistic to suppose the situation was much different in pre-war NHS days but it would need a history of district nursing not written from the viewpoint of the Queen's Institute to investigate this. It is also unclear exactly what sort of nurses were actually being recruited even by the institute. Health visitors needed a fair level of previous education to cope with the examinations set by the Royal Sanitary Institute on behalf of the ministry and could expect secure employment under the favourable conditions of local government employees. District nursing appears to have had lower educational standards and its practitioners were much more likely to end up working in a rather isolated area for a financially precarious voluntary association subject to the whims of its patrons. Stocks, herself, concedes that the remuneration was not much greater than that of a domestic servant and superannuation benefits, in particular, were meagre and begrudged by local associations (Stocks 1960: 160, 162). But perhaps the most conspicuous evidence of district nursing's marginality to health policy is its almost total omission from the official history of the Second World War. Ferguson and Fitzgerald (1954) discuss maternity and child welfare services, tuberculosis care and hospital nursing in exhaustive detail but have virtually nothing to say about district nursing.

Wartime and after

If the contribution of district nurses to the war effort is officially invisible, that of health visitors is reasonably well documented. What is striking, however, is the extent to which health visiting seems to have lost rather than gained ground as a result of this war, in contrast to its experience of 1914–18. This can probably be attributed to the overwhelming pressure on the maternity services.

At the outbreak of war, many clinics were requisitioned for military and civil defence purposes and their health visitors left in place to provide first aid support. This threw a substantial extra burden on the remaining staff which was compounded by the effects of evacuation on the distribution of children. The rural areas which, as we have noted, had always had less developed services found themselves presented not only with the physical and psychological problems associated with evacuation but with new client populations who had much higher expectations about service provision. By 1942, however, the situation had stabilized. The armed services had been barred from further recruitment of health visitors to their nursing services and the numbers of clinics and the rate of home visiting had returned to pre-war levels. The main change, probably reflecting an attempt to get more efficient use of staff, was a growth in local authority employed health visitors at the expense of the voluntary sector (Ferguson and Fitzgerald 1954: 148–53). Figures are not available as full-time equivalents but the voluntary association staff are likely to include a large number of district nurses doing part-time health visiting so that a growth in local authority staff may well indicate a more or less constant amount of time available.

The range of their duties was, however, expanding considerably. From 1943 the ministry was pressing for an increased local authority effort in the care of unmarried mothers and their children. Concern about possible epidemics in 1940 had forced the ministry to abandon its laissez-faire policy on diptheria immunization. In 1937 only about 40 per cent of local authorities had any public scheme and less than 8 per cent of children had been immunized. In the winter of 1940, the ministry agreed to meet all the costs involved and directed authorities to offer immunization, backing this with extensive national and local publicity campaigns. Research in 1942, however, showed that these were less effective than direct personal approaches and the ministry moved to set each health visitor a target of 80 per cent take-up among 1 to 5-year-old children on her caseload. At the end of the war, health visitors were also identified as having a particular part to play in the reintegration of children who had spent long periods in residential nurseries (Ferguson and Fitzgerald 1954: 128–9, 163–7, 248–9).

Table 4 Health visitors employed 1938–46 in England and Wales

	1939	1940	1941	1942	1943	1944	1945	1946
(a)	3,595	3,615	3,654	3,637	3,682	3,716	3,711	3,776
(b)	2,448	2,231	2,160	2,054	2,105	2,229	2,135	2,045
Total	6,043	5,846	5,814	5,691	5,787	5,945	5,846	5,821

(a) Number employed by local authorities
(b) Number employed by voluntary associations

Source: Ferguson and Fitzgerald 1954: 153

But the resources and competence of health visitors to deal with such problems were coming into question. During 1944, health visiting was heavily depleted by the diversion of staff with recent midwifery experience to meet the crisis in the maternity services, a crisis which persisted right through the early years of the NHS. Moreover, there is also evidence that a growing number of social workers were being engaged by local authorities to deal with infant protection, nursery care, and illegitimacy work. By March 1945, for instance, 339 authorities in England and Wales had submitted schemes for the care of unmarried mothers and their children. 210 were in partnership with voluntary organizations and 50 were directed by local authority social workers. The ministry was encouraging the growth of such appointments in preference to arrangements with the voluntary sector (Ferguson and Fitzgerald 1954: 128). The influential *Cambridge Evacuation Survey* directed by Susan Isaacs (1941) and actively supported by John Bowlby makes no reference to a role for health visitors in its discussions of the necessary services for the placement and management of evacuated children. It looks, rather, to the extension of social work appointments at a rate of about 1 per 500 children to permit regular visiting and casework, supported by a psychiatric social work service as a specialist back-up.

The social history of social work is an even less well-tilled field than that of nursing. It is, however, clear that the post-war development of health visiting cannot adequately be understood without a full discussion of developments in social work. The politics of the Children Act 1948 are of particular importance in this. That act followed two important inquiries, that of the Curtis Committee on the Care of Children (HMSO 1946) and the Monckton Report (HMSO 1945) on the death of Denis O'Neil, a child in the care of a local authority. These investigations had pointed to the fragmentation of central and local government responsibilities for children. The Curtis Report proposed the centralization of existing responsibilities in a new children's department of local authorities, which would deal with all children in the care of the state. The Home Office won the struggle with Whitehall for control of the departments. Its inspectorate had experience of social work personnel in the voluntary sector, which had been less heavily criticized by the Curtis Committee, and pressed local authorities to recruit from that pool. But social workers themselves were aspiring to a larger role in the prevention of childhood problems, which rapidly led to tensions between the limited domain of the children's department and the ambitions of the occupation. The competition for this work can be traced through a succession of inquiries and policy debates during the 1950s and 1960s (Packman 1975, Dingwall *et al.* 1984: 224–7). Consideration should probably also be given to the organizational consequences of the nationalization of relief when the Poor Law duties placed upon local authorities in 1929 were centralized by the National Assistance Act 1948 and indeed, the take-over of certain local authority responsibilities by the NHS. Where historians have examined this post-war period, their focus, so far, has tended to be on the new institutions rather than the impact on the old.

The years between 1945 and 1951 saw a major reconstruction of the organization of state health and welfare services. Although maternity services, in particular, continued to be a policy priority, health visiting seems to have lost ground in two directions. It has failed to resist the encroachment of social work in its traditional domain of child welfare and it has failed to colonize the new territories of work in the community with the old, the chronically sick, the handicapped, and the mentally disordered. Since 1945, health visitors have, at various times, been used to provide services in one locality or another to all of these client groups. But in none of them have they actually secured a long-term position as the dominant service provider.

A number of factors seem to be implicated in this. One is the immediate post-war overload from the rising birth rate which seems to have left the specialty short of capacity to cope with any new demands. Indeed the dearth of health visitors and the inability to recruit up to establishments, even where these were large enough to achieve ministry targets, have been endemic problems throughout the post-war years. This constraint almost certainly derives from the general problem of recruitment to nursing, given the fact that the post-war health visiting has been able to draw only on the available pool of registered nurses which has further been restricted by the additional requirement of 5 subjects in School Certificate or GCE 'O' level examinations. It seems unlikely that health visiting could have incorporated new areas of work without breaking the link with nursing. Health visiting was also vulnerable because of its association, fairly or not, with the much criticized history of local authority responsibility for child care. Finally, social work secured a local authority chief officer to speak for it, in the Children's Officer, whereas health visitors were always dependent upon the Medical Officer of Health. Their fate was heavily influenced by the extent of his power in the authority and the degree to which he was motivated to exercise it on their behalf. The Children's Officer had an important ally in the Home Office Inspectorate with its established place in the machinery of government and its leverage on local authorities. Health visiting was a small corner of the responsibilities of the Nursing Division of the Ministry of Health, a newly-formed (1941) group in a large ministry with more pressing concerns.

It would be wrong to imply that there were no attempts to formulate a policy for health visiting. Rather the attempts that were made saw little follow-through or foundered on rival interests. The Jameson Inquiry of 1956 rejected the territorial ambitions of the Royal College of Midwives and the Institute of Almoners and endorsed a broad definition of health visiting as encompassing a good deal of preventive social casework. It also blocked the aspirations of the Queen's Institute to assume a larger role in the aftercare and rehabilitation and called for a sharper distinction between the two specialties in a way which would give the district nurse a subordinate status (Baly 1987: 113–14). But its recommendations were slow to be matched with action. A new Council for the Training of Health Visitors to replace the RSI as the certifying body was set up in close association with the Council for the Training of Social Workers in 1962. However, resources were not forthcoming to match the innovations in education which the CTHV developed. The pace was set by initiatives in social work which led to the establishment of local authority social services departments and the secession of social workers from the association between the two training councils under the Local Authority Social Services Act 1970. The Seebohm Report (HMSO 1968b) was particularly conspicuous in its dismissal of the potential contribution of health visitors and any notion that they should be seen as comparable to social workers dealing with certain clients whose problems were associated with their health status or whose needs were presented in health-related settings. At the same time, health visitors felt profoundly threatened by the recommendations of the Briggs Report (HMSO 1972) which they saw, rightly or wrongly, as overemphasizing the nursing aspects of their work.

If health visiting drifted in a policy vacuum during the post-war period, it is arguable that district nursing has actually fared rather better. This is not necessarily the view of the main historical accounts but these are coloured by their focus on the Queen's Institute which did lose influence. The NHS Act 1946 obliged local authorities to provide a free home nursing service, although the ministry allowed them to continue using voluntary associations as agents for this. Some areas, including East Sussex, Berkshire, Bristol, Liverpool, and Gloucester City continued on this basis. Others including Lancashire, Kent, and Somerset, adopted an intermediate status of being 'in membership' with the institute appointing a Queen's Nurse as superintendent and permitting the institute to inspect their service. Finally, other areas including Durham, Northumberland, Staffordshire, and Glamorgan rejected any link with the institute. The institute retaliated by removing any nurse employed in those areas from its roll (Stocks 1960: 171–9).

While it retained an influence which lingered up to the ending of all agency arrangements with the NHS, in the 1974 reorganization, the institute suffered a decisive defeat on the issue of national training standards. A working party on this question had been set up in parallel to the Jameson Committee's review of health visiting. Its report in 1955 split between a majority who endorsed a four-month training administered by a committee with a strong local authority representation and a minority associated with the Queen's Institute which wanted to adopt the institute's six-month course with itself as the examining body. Despite active lobbying by the institute's supporters, the ministry adopted the majority report. The institute thought that the ministry was more interested in health visitors (Stocks 1960: 199) but it seems more plausible to accept White's (1982) view that, faced with a situation where half the district nurses in the country had no specific training for the work at all, the ministry's main concern was to give as many as possible a minimum level of training as quickly as possible. In effect, the institute's traditional elitism was its own downfall. In the past it had incurred the enmity of a substantial body of local authority opinion. Now its unbending refusal to compromise its ideal standards in the face of the economic and human realities of delivering an acceptable, if not an optimal, service lost it any real influence on the future shape of district nurse training. The London County Council which was, indirectly, the largest employer of Queen's Nurses forced the institute to accept the shorter training with its threat of winding up its agency agreement and making alternative training arrangements. The institute managed to get some detailed modification of the ministry's proposals but when the new national training provisions were announced in 1959, it was clearly to be no more than one among a large number of institutions training nurses for a ministry-administered certificate (Stocks 1960: 192–205). This policy was backed by the Royal College of Nursing which was, at that time, trying to model nursing on medicine with specialist training following a generalist foundation. Unlike medicine, however, the specialist was seen as a team leader rather than an expert provider, which was somewhat at odds with the clinical demands of district work.

As McIntosh (1985) notes, district nurse training did not make much further progress during the 1960s. Nevertheless, as an issue it had been tackled with more urgency than health visitor training and the ministry did attempt to move towards mandatory certification as the supply of trained nurses increased. The introduction of a new curriculum in 1972 was, however, overshadowed by the Briggs Report. District nurses were somewhat less hostile than health visitors but failed to see any great advantage in the reform proposals. These reflected hospital interests which, McIntosh argues, have always undervalued district work because of its low technology content. As she points out, their needs have also tended to be subordinated to those of health visitors in local health service planning. Where they were employed under agency arrangements, local authorities had little incentive to manage them positively. Where they have been directly employed, whether by local authorities or, since 1974, by health authorities, they have usually been grouped into community nursing divisions dominated by health visitor-trained managers. Nevertheless, district nursing has continued to benefit from demographic and policy changes in a way which health visiting has not. But policies are made for district nurses, not by them.

Chapter ten

Professional Autonomy and Economic Constraints

'What experience and history teach is this – that people and governments never have learnt anything from history, or acted on principles deduced from it.' This quotation, from the nineteenth century German philosopher Hegel, is one of the cliches of historical writing. But the statement that people never seem to learn from history is very different from saying that there is nothing to be learnt. The justification for studying history is not only the light it can shed on the roots of present events but its value as data for comparative analyses, taking advantage of some of the theoretical tools provided by other social sciences and their power to explain and to predict. It may be true that one can never cross the same river twice but a knowledge of winds, rocks and currents is still likely to lead to a safer passage.

This final chapter, then, is located in that ill-defined space where sociology, economics and the other social sciences of the present merge into history, the social science of the past. It looks at events in nursing since the Briggs Committee was set up in 1970 as part of a long process of occupational development. It uses the analysis constructed in the course of the preceding pages to explore structural and cultural changes as diverse as the Griffiths reorganization, Project 2000 and the spread of the nursing process. In particular, it examines the continuing struggle between managerial and professional versions of the occupation, contrasting the utilitarian emphasis on service provision with the attempts to 'gentrify' the property. It concludes with an evaluation of the prospects for nursing in the light of the fundamental economic and social constraints which have been identified.

The Briggs Committee

We observed at the end of Chapter 6 (p. 113) that the Briggs

Committee was set up against a background of industrial unrest. In this respect it resembled most of the major policy initiatives in nursing since the Nurses Registration Act 1919. Indeed, looking at the politics of the act itself and of the subsequent Athlone and Wood committees, it is difficult to resist the conclusion that central government's standard approach to questions of nursing policy is one of crisis management.

The diaries left by Richard Crossman, the then Secretary of State for Social Services, clearly establish that his prime motive in setting up the Briggs Committee was to relieve the government's embarrassment over the threat posed by nurses to its prices and incomes policy. The challenge took the form both of direct industrial action and the quieter protest of high rates of wastage and turnover. This diary entry is dated 23 December 1969:

> We've got to make an offer which is not derisory but that means it will go beyond 4 per cent and break Barbara's prices and incomes policy.[1] I think we can only get away with this by saying nurses are low-paid workers and that we must give them a completely new standing and a new pay structure. I have also persuaded Asa Briggs to undertake a special investigation of this. (Crossman 1977: 759)

But, as with the Registration Act itself and the Wood inquiry, the Briggs Committee also needs to be examined in the context of plans for reorganizing the health services as a whole. A further and unique element in the early 1970s was the progress of a general and relatively non-partisan programme for modernizing the legislation regulating a number of professions, including medicine and dentistry.

Unlike the Wood Committee, Briggs was not given a free hand to reconstruct nursing to meet the needs of the reorganized service. While both had been set up at a point where the government was committed to structural change in the delivery of health care, Wood had been invited to calculate staffing and training requirements from scratch (Ministry of Health 1947:1): Briggs, on the other hand, was directed to plan within existing 'manpower' constraints (HMSO 1972: 1). A good deal of the committee's energy was absorbed by detailed investigations of the potential supply and demand for labour in nursing and of patterns of wastage and turnover. But the committee seems to have been reluctant to go on to examine the cost implications of its proposals, beyond acknowledging that they would be 'substantial'. It devoted barely two pages to a discussion of this topic. For all the economic advice available to it, the committee made no attempt to quantify the costs or benefits of change and merely asserted the positive economic returns to be expected (HMSO 1972: 193–5). This may well reflect a political judgement of the desirability of avoiding any recommendation that would obviously entail increased public expenditure in the difficult economic climate of the early 1970s. But once such critical managerial concerns had been ruled out of order the committee inevitably found itself with a vague agenda. It became a place where the occupation could ventilate its grievances rather than for planning serious change. As such, it was typical of many of the Royal Commissions and Departmental Committees which were used by the 1964–70 Labour Government to deflect short-term political problems.

This background is important to understanding both the nature of the committee's deliberations and the fate of its report. Once new investment was ruled out, managerial interests could disengage themselves from the committee's work, in the knowledge that its proposals could always be modified in their implementation by playing the 'resource implications' card. Indeed, the committee's recommendations on management are little more than platitudes (HMSO 1972: 168–70). The field, then, was left clear for the professionalizing segment of the occupation to gain control of the committee's deliberations. The importance of the clash between 'professional' and 'managerial' interests in shaping the educational experience of student nurses has been demonstrated at the level of practice by Melia (1984, 1987).

It is equally relevant to the analysis of educational policy. Dingwall (1974) has previously shown that many of the experiments in education during the late 1950s and early 1960s could be seen as part of a strategy of professionalization by certain segments of the occupation. In this book we have shown that its roots lie deep in the nineteenth century and the aspiration to create new careers for educated women. These contemporary developments were not socially neutral but were an attempt to protect or enlarge nursing's share of the market for well-qualified and, almost inevitably, middle-class girl school leavers. As in the 1930s, they are important evidence of the occupational image which the leadership, or at least a section of it, wanted to create. This tendency is one of the most conspicuous features of the Briggs Report. Its thinking starts from the poor image of the occupation among school leavers and the particular failure to compete with higher education for those with 2 'A' levels, although this is embedded in fashionable rhetoric about the need to encourage mature entrants (HMSO 1972: 54, 61, 83, 98–9). The remedy lies in a direct line of descent from Mrs Bedford Fenwick's proposals for a nursing curriculum structured along medical lines, with a general foundation leading on to specialist qualifications.

The actual recommendations were not, of course, literal recapitulations of the ideas of the 1920s. They were also coloured by the educational fashions of the time. Wood, for example, had been preoccupied with the use of intelligence tests to predict the educability of potential entrants. The same thinking dominated the implementation of the Education Act 1944 and produced the tripartite classification of secondary schools into grammar, technical and secondary modern (Evans 1975: 109–10). Briggs, on the other hand, offered a 'comprehensive' vision of nursing education, with each individual being free to select the track and pace of learning which suited them. The new training would foster 'mixed ability' intake on to a common programme. This would be organized on the basis of learning modules, discrete blocks of knowledge which could be repeated until mastered. Everyone could succeed at something.

Within this apparently egalitarian system, however, an elaborate meritocracy would be created. The initial 18-month programme would lead to a Certificate, but a further 18 months' study would be required for Registration and selected candidates would be able to continue to a Higher Certificate after that (HMSO 1972: 85–94). Graduate programmes would be left largely outside this structure, although they were seen as the main source of professional leadership for the future (HMSO 1972: 96–7). The proposed content of the training reformulated the old objective of integrating curative and preventive work, an ideal which certainly goes back to Florence Nightingale and her suspicion of hospitals but which had been restated both by the GNC in the early 1920s and by the Wood Committee.

To oversee the system, Briggs proposed the consolidation of the various bodies responsible for overseeing pre- and post-registration training in the various specialties and parts of the United Kingdom. The result would be a single, powerful council supported by national boards charged with the implementation of its policies on education and discipline. All the various sections of the occupation would be brought under its governance. The only specialty to retain any degree of autonomy would be midwifery, which would be regulated by a statutory committee of the Council (HMSO 1972: 185–90). It seemed like a final victory for the assimilationists.

But the victory was a hollow one. The committee had been set up under a Labour government and only narrowly avoided being terminated prematurely when the Conservatives took office in

1970. The new minister, Sir Keith Joseph, had no particular commitment to the review or its report, but, rather than rejecting it outright, he initiated the first in a protracted series of consultation exercises. It was only in 1974, following another change of government, that Barbara Castle, now the Labour Secretary of State for Social Services, announced the acceptance of the committee's main recommendations. But this statement was itself made against the background of further industrial unrest within the occupation, which was eventually bought off only by the offer of an independent inquiry into pay and conditions. This review, chaired by the Earl of Halsbury, awarded increases in pay of up to 40 per cent. The cost implications for the NHS were enormous: each 1 per cent increase in nurses' pay represents about £35 million on the pay bill. Moreover, the review body also stated that its conclusions and recommendations assumed the implementation of the Briggs proposals with all the expenditure that they implied. Action on Briggs had been stalled by the appointment of the Halsbury review: it now returned to the policy agenda. In the autumn of 1974 the DHSS responded in classic civil service fashion by setting up another period of consultation, which eventually led to the formation of a Briggs Co-ordinating Committee in 1977. This brought departmental officials together with representatives of the nursing organizations to discuss the necessary legislative change. A bill was finally introduced into what was widely expected to be the last session of the parliament in November 1978.

There were important similarities between the objectives of the bill and of the Nurses Registration Act 1919. Both were concerned with standards and mobility within the occupation and attempted to create structures that would encourage greater occupational unity. They endeavoured to bring order to what Celia Davies (1985: 36) has called the 'patchwork quilt' of nurse education. When the bill was published, however, it proved a bitter disappointment to its sponsors within nursing. It concentrated almost entirely on the reform of the regulatory structure and gave virtually no attention to the educational questions which had so preoccupied the professionalist segment of the occupation. The DHSS interpretation of 'main recommendations' proved to refer to the council and boards alone. Dr Gerard Vaughan, Conservative MP for Reading South, compared the bill to the Cheshire Cat from Alice in Wonderland:

> It is all smiles, it is all head, perhaps it is all brains, but there is no body to it. (*House of Commons Debates*, 1978 13 Nov. col. 55)

In his view, it made no contribution to solving the critical problems of staff shortages, inadequate pay and falling standards of care. It would 'do nothing to put right the industrial unrest and in some cases unemployment among nurses' (ibid., col. 57). Like the Nurses Registration Act 1919, it seems as though the Nurses, Midwives and Health Visitors Bill was to be confined to the 'smallest possible compass'.

Why were the professionalizers' expectations so quickly disappointed? In part, it may well be because they were inflated by their interpretation of the Briggs Report. Reading it after a lapse of time, it is striking how much attention is given to structural details and how little to any discussion of the fundamental nature of nursing work. Where this does occur it merely recapitulates the position of the professionalizers. For example, the possible development of some nurses as treatment assistants is simply dismissed as not fitting into the health pattern of this country (HMSO 1972: 47). As we have shown, this view is, to say the least, unconscious of the historical evidence. Moreover it denies to nurses the job satisfaction of practitioner roles, as these were developing in the USA in the early 1970s and have continued to extend since. What it does do is to insist on a view of nursing as separate from but equal to the medical profession. Where others work or perform tasks, nursing cares and coordinates: 'Nursing and midwifery is more than a workforce. It is a profession.' (HMSO 1972: 158).

In the same way, the text of the report gives a marginal place to nursing in research and higher education. The main proposal for educational reform was the creation of colleges of health, grouping nurses with other paramedical occupations in an institution somewhere between a teacher training college and a college of further education. Only 2 to 5 per cent of the occupation should be recruited through higher education (HMSO 1972: 96–7, 107–8). This elite would have a particular role to play in research, in association with specialists in social or life sciences. The celebrated line about nursing becoming a 'research-based profession' is followed by the observation that 'as in other professions, the active pursuit of serious research must be limited to a minority'. All Briggs actually advocates is that 'a sense of the need for research should become part of the mental equipment of every practising nurse or midwife' (HMSO 1972: 108).

If the advocates of professionalization had overestimated the support which they could derive from the text of the Briggs Report, they had also underestimated the extent to which their own occupation was united behind the demands for change. As in

1919 various specialist interests feared that the concentration of power would inevitably lead to the practical and ideological dominance of general hospital nursing. This time the main opposition came from health visitors and midwives. The health visitors were particularly concerned by the threat to their existing integration with mainstream further and higher education posed by the Briggs proposals to unify all nurse education in independent colleges. They believed, probably correctly, that such institutions were likely to lack academic credibility and to fail to attract the other paramedical groups who were actively developing their own polytechnic and university based programmes. As with the major hospitals in 1919 which had already developed advanced training provision, they feared that the consequence of unification would be to level down standards and devalue their qualifications. They doubted whether their commitment to preventive work would survive without a more distinctive base than a few modules in a clinically oriented training.

Some midwives supported the changes but an important section saw them as a further move towards reducing their status to that of maternity nurses and abandoning any claim to a practitioner role. There is less evidence on this occasion of serious opposition from the mental nursing sectors, possibly because they had already been more fully absorbed by the GNC. Although Briggs again dismissed the claim of paid carers for the mentally handicapped to a legitimate place in the occupation, their attention was diverted to the struggle for the ear of the Jay Committee rather than the new regulatory legislation.

To some extent, the occupational leadership was also divided on national lines. The Kilbrandon Commission had recommended the establishment of a Scottish Assembly in 1973 which would, among other things, assume responsibility for Scottish health services. Although its proposals were never implemented, the currents of concern about devolution were running so strongly in the 1970s that the Scots were not pleased to see their autonomous GNC replaced by a national board that would be subordinate to a UK council which would inevitably be dominated by the numerical weight of English interests. This is again reminiscent of 1919 and the concern of the Scots over the fate of their established system of certification.

These various interests succeeded in getting some significant changes to the original Briggs proposals. The health visitors moved towards parity with the midwives by obtaining their own statutory committee, although its powers were more limited and its practical status ambiguous. The idea of setting up new colleges was dropped, although this probably owed more to the potential cost and the change in educational fashion away from small monotechnic institutions which was leading to the closure of many teacher training colleges and the amalgamation of others with polytechnics. The devolutionists succeeded in strengthening the powers of the boards at the expense of the council.

The DHSS also had its own priorities. Throughout the 1970s it was preoccupied by successive reorganizations of the NHS. Although some of the recommendations of the Briggs Committee were in line with its own attempts to achieve a closer integration of hospital and community based health services, the reform of nursing was less urgent than the development of the new management structures. Given the extent to which they have since been criticized, it is important to recall the original objectives. The reforms were motivated by exactly the same concerns as the Griffiths reorganization of the 1980s, namely the desire to achieve a more effective and efficient use of human and physical resources. The large measure of autonomy left to regional boards and hospital management committees in 1948 was seen as an obstacle. Regional boards were too remote and HMCs too small to support comprehensive management services. As a result decision-making reflected the outcome of local clinical politicking rather than any sort of rational plan. The teaching hospitals were not even part of the system at all. Moreover, the division of responsibility between NHS and local authority health services was seen as a source of waste, duplication and gaps in coverage.

In keeping with the contemporary fashion in management theory, it was thought that the reformers' goals could be achieved by a combination of central planning and bureaucratization.[2] The 1960s and 1970s were a period of great faith in the value of bringing interest groups together in order to agree on the objectives of an organization on any scale, from an individual factory to the whole country. This agreement would be set down in a plan which the partners would then attempt to implement. In such a system, management became very much a matter of administration, executing the agreed programme rather than taking independent initiatives. Given the peculiar complexity of the producer interests in the NHS, a collegial form of bureaucracy was adopted in the guise of 'consensus management'. Representatives of all the major professional groups were invited to join with the administrators in developing rational plans which each would then impose on its own members.

Potentially, nursing stood to gain a great deal from this. Part of the objective was to bring collegial pressure to bear on the apparently unregulated growth of medical expenditure. Nurses could have been key allies of the administrators in this process, both in identifying lower-cost solutions, possibly involving the substitution of nursing for medical labour, and in monitoring the knock-on effects of medical decisions. A new consultant means new procedures, more nurses, more drugs, etc. All of these need to be costed in with the decision to create the post rather than treating it simply as a matter for the medical staff budget. Certainly the structure gave nurses a more central place in hospital decision-making than they had ever enjoyed. It was not just matron having direct access to the board of governors: nurse managers now had a guaranteed seat on every major committee as an integral part of the consensus management team.

In practice, however, the opportunity was lost. A number of factors were involved in this. Some were beyond the scope of nursing to influence, like the resistance of the medical profession to any kind of collective responsibility which meant that they could never be relied on to honour agreements made by their represent-atives in the management process. Others, however, reflected the undervaluation of the management function in nursing itself. Many of the nurse managers were inevitably people already in post under a very different system. They were asked to transform their approach and to adopt new techniques and collective goals with very little retraining. The network of committees that was created to give them professional advice proved only how few nurses had sufficient education to grasp the critical issues of service policy and planning (Robinson and Strong 1987: 22–9). Within their own occupation they became the butt of the professionalizers' criticism for their obstruction of the development of autonomous practice by registered nurses.

But such a goal was quite antithetical to the objectives of the change. The point was that it was not clear that the NHS, or, indeed, any other developed health care system, could afford one autonomous, free-spending profession, let alone two. Thus, the traditions of hierarchy and obedience which had been introduced by the Victorians to manage their nurse–servants were transformed into a more modern industrial discipline. It left the private life and character of the nurse to one side. She was no longer likely to be struck off for having illegitimate children, living in adulterous relationships or going to hotels with men (Pyne 1981: 20–6). Now her loyalty lay only to the plans which her line managers had helped to devise. There was no place for the highly individualized judgement of the professional and little support for educational changes that could destabilize the relationship between manage-

212

ment and ward-level staff. In reality, nurse management was intended more as a model for the organization of medicine than vice versa.

It is also important to recognize the internal policy agenda of the civil servants in the DHSS. During the 1970s, the regulatory framework for a number of health professions was reviewed and modernized.[3] Although this provoked a good deal of debate within the professions affected, it was not treated as a particularly partisan matter and proceeded almost regardless of which government was in office. Indeed, it can be argued that a similar kind of reform might well have occurred as a civil service initiative, whether or not the Briggs Committee had ever been appointed. The DHSS simply took advantage of a move originally conditioned by political expediency. From a civil service point of view, the 1970s were a favourable period for carrying out this kind of legislative housekeeping because the absence of a clear majority for either party during most of the decade meant that it was difficult to fill parliamentary time with controversial bills. These measures of professional reform represent the kind of proposals which any department could keep on the shelf until an opportunity appeared. In this case, it was a parliamentary session when an election was expected but the government was anxious to avoid being forced into a premature move by defeat on a major item of its programme.

In the light of these various considerations, the professionalizers' disappointment with the Nurses, Midwives and Health Visitors Act 1979 becomes easier to understand. Instead of the construction of a new licence for autonomous practice, they were presented with a low-cost administrative reform whose concessions to a number of special interests limited their ability to impose a unified view of the occupation's status and direction.

The nursing process

Melia (1984, 1987) has pointed out that the professionalizers' main base in nursing lies in the educational sector, among people who do not have a day-to-day responsibility for service provision. Their response to the rejection of their version of the Briggs recommendations was to use the institutions which they did control more aggressively to impose a professional ideal on new entrants or those who passed through in pursuit of advanced training. One of the major vehicles for this was the nursing process.

The history of the nursing process has been analysed in some detail by de la Cuesta (1983). As she points out, this approach to nursing work developed during the late 1950s and 1960s in the United States primarily for teaching purposes. It was a useful method of helping experienced nurses to think more systematically about their practice while on courses intended to update their original training. Although a few hospitals experimented with it as a system for the organization of care, it made little impact on practice until the 1970s when the Joint Commission on the Accreditation of Hospitals, which certifies the quality of hospital services as a basis for Federal and private insurance payments, made the preparation of care plans a prerequisite for its approval of an institution.

De la Cuesta does not bring out the full significance of this decision and the implications of the nursing process being imposed as a management tool but it is of considerable significance to her arguments about its transformation in the UK. Care plans became one of the book-keeping devices by which American health planners tried to contain the escalating costs of medical care. They required each item of nursing service to be identified and justified. If an item was not clearly related to the plan or accepted by later reviewers the hospital might be denied reimbursement for its costs. The preparation of such documents became a considerable administrative art in itself (Gubrium 1980, Gubrium and Buckholdt 1982: 127–71, Gubrium 1975: 39–82).

The nursing process as such first began to be discussed in Britain during 1973 although no articles were published on the subject until 1975. It remained a topic for discussion within a narrow circle until it suddenly appeared in the syllabus for general nurse training in 1977.[4] De la Cuesta notes the transformation which occurred in its passage across the Atlantic. The American emphasis on intellectual skills and the individual accountability of the nurse was played down as was any notion of care planning being an exercise in which the patient would be an active participant. The nursing process was represented as a means of remedying certain complaints by nurses rather than directly addressing the needs of patients.

In her review of nursing literature from Britain in the early 1970s, de la Cuesta identifies a set of related dissatisfactions with the way nursing work was organized. These focused on the way patient care was broken down into a set of tasks so that the nurse's experience of the work was fragmented and the patient was treated as a collection of unit tasks rather than as a whole person. From the nurses' point of view, this encouraged superficial nurse/patient relationships which they found unrewarding. The nursing process promised to change all this by matching patients and nurses as individuals and integrating task performance into a varied series of services performed by one person for another. It was the latest in a number of attempts to alter the pattern of ward organization which had previously been based on more partial concepts such as patient-centred care, patient assignment and team nursing.

While the nursing process has been successfully imposed on the syllabi for most areas of nurse education, with the exception of midwifery, the impact on practice has been almost universally disappointing. The *Report of the Nursing Process Evaluation Group* organized by the Nursing Education Research Unit at King's College, London for the DHSS (Hayward 1986) reviewed most of the available studies and collected opinion from a variety of sources. The group could find very few examples of successful implementation. They concluded by calling for more extensive education and consultation in advance of change. This, of course, is a traditional explanation for organizational failure – blaming the ignorance or incapacity of lower-level personnel rather than examining the features of the system which made it possible for the breakdown to occur.[5]

De la Cuesta reached a similarly pessimistic conclusion about the introduction of the nursing process from interviews and observation in both British and American hospitals which made some claim to have adopted it as a method of working. While nursing histories were widely used, they were treated as reference sheets rather than as the foundation for a nursing diagnosis and a care plan. Care plans were inconsistently written and emphasized the medical care of patients and the physical tasks which the nurses would need to perform. Unlike the King's College Group, however, who, interestingly, do not cite her work, de la Cuesta goes on to search for the organizational reasons for the lack of enthusiasm among ward staff. She points out that these are additional burdens of paperwork on busy staff. Although they may be idealized by nursing theorists, they represent work which is not symbolically valued by the hospital. The records are destroyed when patients are discharged. Staff allocations still demonstrate a priority for physical care: when demands for this are lowest, in the afternoons, staffing levels are reduced rather than allowing extra time for psycho-social work. If a nurse does commit her plans to paper, then she is likely to become accountable for them. The prevailing experience of nurses is that good work does not bring rewards but poor work or failure to meet a set target is certainly likely to incur sanctions. A more intense individual involvement with patients creates a greater risk of emotional stress on the nurse.

This last observation suggests a possible linkage to much more fundamental analyses of the conditions generating the present pattern of ward organization. Menzies (1963) argued that task splitting was an important form of psychological self-defence for nurses. If responsibility was diffused or shared the impact of the inevitable failure of all nursing care was diluted. However good a health care system, all patients ultimately die. Although there is some evidence that the nursing process can increase job satisfaction (e.g. Bowman *et al.* 1983), this tends to come from pilot schemes and may well represent a Hawthorne effect, i.e. the satisfaction may be caused by the attention paid to staff in the course of the experiment rather than deriving from the changes themselves.[6]

More recently, Melia (1987) has brought out the organizational logic of task allocation. It is a rational response to the economic pressures which hospitals have experienced for at least the last hundred years. Task allocation is a way of organizing work into blocks which are capable of being performed by anyone of a given skill level. When general nurse training was reorganized in the nineteenth century to dilute loyalty to particular wards and encourage loyalty to the occupation, the cheapest form of labour, trainees, also became mobile. A ward sister could not be certain of the individual competence of whichever of the students happened to be assigned to her ward on a given day. She resolved this by structuring the work to be done on the basis of predetermined slots or roles into which any student at a particular stage of her training could be inserted.

The nursing process, in itself, does nothing to alter these environmental features of nursing practice. It therefore seems implausible to attribute the poor results of implementation programmes solely to a lack of education on the part of the participants. These programmes may fail because they do not take account of the real conditions of nursing work. De la Cuesta herself concludes by arguing that the nursing process must be understood as an ideology as much as a practice. It is a body of ideas which responds to the problems of a particular time rather than being spontaneously generated. Viewed in these terms, the nursing process could be seen to have three aspects, depending upon whether one takes the perspective of its advocates, of patients, or of health service administrators.

A good place to begin examining the professionalizers' perspective is the question of job satisfaction. Why was there a sudden revolt against task-based patient care in the 1960s? Two possible explanations come to mind. One would be that it reflects wider social movements in that decade which were based on a call for more holistic relationships between people than modern societies seem to offer. It was a rejection of 'one-dimensional' views of humanity. The other explanation would reflect the status anxieties of the traditional nursing elite which, it was suggested above, gave rise to the educational experiments of the period. They reformulated the idea of professionalism in nursing using terms which were derived from private practice. One of the big problems for the sociological analyst of professions is the way definitions, especially from North America, build in implicit assumptions about a private relationship between professional and client. In nursing, those same assumptions come through in the proposal that the ideal relationship is that of an individual nurse to an individual patient. Managers, health care planners, and the state are all unnecessary impediments. Thus, task allocation comes to be seen as a problem, as unworthy of a true profession.

To the extent that American nursing was seen as more prestigious than British in the 1960s, because of its more rapid expansion of graduate programmes, under the very different conditions of a society committed to a mass system of higher education, and its apparently greater economic success, its practices represented a model for ambitious British nurses. More exactly, the model was those practices which were documented in print or carried by nurses in education with the opportunity and resources to travel.

The nursing process came from a well-regarded source and expressed the solution to the status grievances which had been articulated. Indeed much of its language – the nursing diagnosis and the nursing prescription for care – borrowed directly from medicine just as Mrs Bedford Fenwick had.

Having captured the language of professionalism it could be used to impose an ideological hegemony on other sections of the occupation. General nursing and some closely related sections of district nursing were almost certainly the areas which felt the keenest sense of loss from nationalization. Midwifery was threatened by other social and technical changes, mental nursing had always been carried out mostly in public sector institutions by nurses who saw themselves as part of a manual workforce and health visiting was virtually untouched, remaining part of local government until 1974. The nursing process could be used to impose a common occupational culture, dominated by general nursing, an aspiration which certainly went back to the original registration debates. So, we can trace the demands for a mental nursing process, a midwifery process, a health visiting process and so on. As the

King's College Group Report shows, the success has been uneven in terms of practice, but quite considerable in terms of syllabi for training.

In some segments of the occupation, the results would introduce a major transformation. This is perhaps most obvious in the case of health visiting, which is founded on a quite different philosophy. Systematic approaches are not new in health visiting. The language of objectives formed an integral part of health visitor courses in the early 1970s, although it was then derived from educational theory. But, as the CETHV (1977, 1980, 1982) saw in some of its last documents before being absorbed into the new structure, the essence of health visiting has always been the search for health needs. Routine home visiting was an integral part of this, as a means for identifying unrecognized need. Its legitimation derived from the national interest in the early detection and remedy of incipient cases of disease or handicap. Health visiting is essentially about the surveillance of the private space of people's lives. There is nothing intrinsically wrong with this but the general ideological climate of the times is unfavourable to such surveillance, although demanding it vigorously in particular instances, such as cases of child abuse (Dingwall *et al.* 1983). Process approaches in health visiting roll with this tide by switching the emphasis away from the routine visit to clinic-based work which responds to need expressed in terms defined in advance by the health visitor.[7] A service will be offered which clients may or may not use as they wish. While it may well be arguable that a great deal of home visiting has been done in a fairly unsystematic way and that it should not be uncritically defended, it is important to recognize the radical nature of the changes that are being proposed.

This point can be explored further if we consider the responses of patients. The King's College Group conceded that very little is known about the way patients react to this approach to their care, a gap in the research which further supports our earlier contention that the nursing process has been driven by the desire to solve nurses' problems rather than to respond to those of patients. The group cite Brooking's (1986) doctoral thesis to the effect that process-based nursing demands that patients take a more active role in their own care. She found, however, that the majority of patients saw their role as essentially passive. This finding is in line with the Fitton and Acheson (1979) study of patient responses to different styles of general practice. Working-class patients, in particular, preferred to deal with doctors on a technical level, what has elsewhere been called the car mechanic's model. If they were ill, they wanted to be fixed up rather than to be subjected to what they regarded as intrusive personal inquiries. Indeed, this response is very much in line with what might be predicted on theoretical grounds from Parsons's (1952) analysis of the sick role, which emphasizes patient compliance with expert prescriptions rather than self-directed actions. It may well be significant that the greatest advance of process nursing is in the care of client groups like the elderly who are least well-placed to resist its encroachments.

What the nursing process and its analogues in medicine like Balint-style general practice share is the way they implicate patients' psyches in the outcome of their treatment. If we recall our discussion of social control in Chapter 2, we can identify them as part of a new strategy. Disease was first a matter for small economic groups. The creation of an integrated national economy made it a national concern. This was first expressed in the segregation of the sick in hospitals, workhouses and asylums. It was extended into the home with the growth of social forms of medicine. Now, as Armstrong (1983) and Silverman (1987) discuss, it seeks to penetrate the personality of the patient. The roots of disease lie in disordered life-choices. The mistaken grounds of these choices must be exposed and corrected by psychosocial inquiry.

In some ways, this approach is reminiscent of the philosophy of the Charity Organization Society in its linkage of personal failure to social deviance, in this case sickness. It is not, of course, identical because of its location in a public agency rather than a private charity. But it provides a defensible strategy for service providers trying to cope with a chronic shortage of resources. The COS tests could be seen as a device for rationing relief in the face of overwhelming need and great social instability. The nursing process could be used to deny resources to all but those who show their compliance with a desired moral order. Only those who seek help on terms defined by the care providers, or who will accept their prescriptions to the letter, will receive aid. But the care providers themselves will be exonerated from the burden of choice: those who do not receive aid have only themselves to blame. It is their own decisions which have led them to their predicament and they cannot expect others to bale them out.

From a managerial perspective, the nursing process is a mixed blessing. The cost implications of the professionalization of nursing are certainly unwelcome. In an era when all advanced societies are struggling to contain the economic consequences of medical autonomy, it is unlikely that nursing will make much real progress in that direction. However, as Freidson (1970b: 22) has pointed out, an encouragement of professional work values can be advantageous to employers. By focusing on the needs of individuals, the nursing process encourages an identification between the nurse and the patient. Again it is the model of private practice where the patient's trust in an individual professional is matched by the professional's personal loyalty to him. As Strong (1979, 1988, Strong and Davis 1977) has shown, this is very different from the usual form of patient/practitioner encounter in the NHS, which he describes as 'bureaucratic'. By this, he means that the parties confront each other as instances of a type rather than as people with any particular personal involvement in the interaction. Each is relatively anonymous and their exchanges centre on the clinical task at hand rather than introducing other dimensions of their lives. The commercial impetus, however, gives a quite different shape to private consultations. Here the practitioner may attempt to retain the patient's custom by trying to create a longer-term relationship, independent of any particular contact, to which both sides are personally committed. To the extent that more of the patient's self is engaged, the opportunities for influencing behaviour may be increased.

But this individualization of the relationship is not only a way of disciplining the patient: it can also be a way of disciplining the nurse. Any attempt to pursue her own interest in the organization becomes a breach of trust. In this way the nursing process can be used to divide nurses from each other and to erode their commitment to any industrial goal. Personal objectives are confused with those of the occupation or the organization. The recent proposals for 'primary nursing' represent the most logical extreme of this movement.

A further attraction of the nursing process from a managerial perspective is the volume of paper which it generates. We have already noted this as a feature of the spread of this approach in the United States. It can be held up as an important tool for quality assurance programmes (Dickson 1987: 25–8, Hayward 1986: 25, Pearson 1983: 82–96). But, as de la Cuesta (1983) hints, this also gives it a significant potential for accounting control of nursing. Paradoxically, the individualization of care when coupled with its elaborate documentation can actually increase the scope for external influences, not by direct intervention or instruction but by the setting of norms, standards or targets. The nursing process opens the doors for the development of nursing equivalents of diagnosis related groups, the standard care packages which are used in the United States as the basis of insurance reimbursement. A given disorder is rated at a fixed cost: the hospital and physician must beat that if they are to show a profit, whatever the individual circumstances of the case. The ratings reflect the detailed analysis of the work performed by providers judged by insurers to be efficient. By creating such a detailed analysis of care work, the nursing process not only encourages such evaluations but also gives managers an opportunity to review the mix of staff employed and to consider the extent to which it can be diluted in the search for economy.

The reference to the control of staff by targets or incentives introduces another type of discipline which we shall discuss shortly. For the present, however, it should perhaps be stressed that we should not be read as criticizing the desirability of systematic approaches to nursing care, individual attention to patients or efficient management of health services. The point is, as de la Cuesta (1983) observed, that the attempts to achieve these objectives occur in a particular historical context and the form which they take reflects those general conditions. In that sense it is important to understand the politics of the nursing process, both in terms of a struggle within nursing and in terms of a wider reconstruction of the welfare state.

Griffiths and Project 2000

The most recent phase of the contest between managerial and professional versions of nursing can be examined through two important groups of documents. On the one hand, there are the various publications inspired by the Griffiths Inquiry into NHS Management (DHSS 1983) which set out a new philosophy for NHS administration. On the other, a cluster of reports directed to the reform of nursing education for the twenty-first century.

As we commented earlier, the NHS reorganization of the 1970s had occurred in a political and cultural environment favourable to the concept of collaboration between management and employees in the planning and operation of private and public services. This tended to define management as the administration of an agreed programme rather than as a source of independent initiative. By the 1980s fashions had changed. It was now argued that this resulted in a conservative and inefficient approach to production which featherbedded both managers and workers while neglecting the wishes of consumers. This was expressed in such phenomena as the desertion of public for private provision, the problems of sustaining large-scale enterprises such as the motor industry and the preference of private purchasers for imported consumer goods. If British industry and services were to become internationally competitive again they must become more market-oriented, giving people what they wanted rather than what it suited the producers to provide. This demanded faster responses to changing market conditions than the cumbersome processes which consensus management could achieve. One area of British enterprise which was seen to have been conspicuously successful in this was retailing. So Derek Rayner was brought from Marks and Spencer to review the civil service and Roy Griffiths came from Sainsbury's to examine the NHS.

These exercises brought with them an overdue concern for establishing what things cost – the use of space, the labour inputs, goods and services bought in or supplied internally – and a different conception of management. The emphasis now was on speed and decisiveness rather than on the building of consensus prior to action. As the slogan had it, management's job was to manage. Everyone else merely had to fall into line. Just as importantly, managers were no longer to be bound by detailed regulations. They were to be set targets for their performance, and rewarded or penalized to the extent that they succeeded or failed in meeting them, but the methods which they should adopt were not to be prescribed in detail. It was believed that this would give more scope for innovation and adaptation to local circumstances and needs. A rigid central financial control would be balanced by peripheral organizational flexibility.

In practice this model of the NHS as a holding company, with a small group of accountants at HQ monitoring the financial performance of the division or plants, has proved difficult to reconcile with the demands of public accountability. These impose many constraints from Treasury rules on expenditure to the restriction of the right to prescribe to appropriately licensed persons. The margin in which any NHS manager can effect change is surprisingly small. These built-in inflexibilities have been compounded by the persistent squeeze on resources. The DHSS's assumptions about efficiency savings have clawed back any productivity improvement rather than making the funds available for reinvestment. Thus there has been relatively little scope, for example, to increase the amount of capital per employee and to continue making productivity gains.

Against this background, the managers' interest in nursing reform becomes intelligible. Nursing salaries are one of the largest single items of public expenditure in the UK, consuming almost 3 per cent of the total. Even a small proportional saving could have a large absolute impact. Conversely, any change proposed by the occupation is likely to be assessed carefully for its cost implications.

The professionalizers within nursing have certainly encouraged this interest by their own continuing campaign for educational reform. This was renewed in three documents published during 1985–6 by the English National Board (1985), the RCN (1985) and the UKCC (1986). Somewhat to the private irritation of the UKCC, its Project 2000 review of nursing education was upstaged by the ENB Report. The board's scope for this move reflects the shift between Briggs and the 1979 Act and the greater powers devolved to them. It allowed the professional interests, who had a stronger grip there and more resources available than in the other boards, to set the agenda for the debates.

The ENB proposals were concerned mainly with educational objectives and curriculum content, which were clearly within their powers. In renewing the Bedford Fenwick call for a general foundation programme for all nurses, however, they were clearly spilling on to UKCC turf. Their advocacy of a base in higher education for all nurse training was echoed by the RCN report, from a committee chaired by Sir Harry Judge, director of educational studies at Oxford University, and containing a heavy weighting of higher educationalists. It may not be entirely coincidental that the sudden rise in goodwill towards nurses from higher education coincided with the latter's own straitened financial circumstances. These documents did much to prepare the ground for the UKCC report which also advocated a common core and closer links to higher education. In a later (1987) report from Project 2000, the UKCC strengthened the analogy with medical education even more by calling for the development of certified specialist practitioners who would occupy a distinct clinical career grade as consultants to other nurses.

The arguments for change were made somewhat differently in the various reports. The ENB simply take its desirability for granted, while the RCN Commission, as might be expected from its membership, concentrates on the general desirability of more education. Both tend to emphasize the benefits to nurses rather than discussing standards of care or patient welfare. The UKCC team, however, does attempt to start from an appraisal of the likely pattern of need in hospitals and in the community and only then discusses how this might be met. Moreover, it is the only report to present a number of options for discussion, although its own preferences are quite clear.

There is at least one rather paradoxical implication of all these developments, namely a possible weakening of professional control over the basic curriculum. The ENB's conception of the core, for example, reveals little in the way of specifically nursing content. Although this is understandable in terms of the need to devise a programme at a high level of generalization so as to cover the varied tasks owned by the different segments of the occupation, it reduces the need for nursing experience in teaching the programme. It is possible that the professionalizers hope that it may be possible to impose the sort of closure achieved by schoolteaching and social work, where the professional qualification may be more important than subject knowledge as a credential.

However, the climate in which the terms of entry to higher education are being negotiated is very different and the pool of available staff more limited. If institutions of higher education see nursing courses as a way of employing surplus staff and relatively few nurse tutors have the graduate credentials that would make them acceptable to the institutions, it is not difficult to envisage a situation where qualified nurses are marginalized in nurse education. They may teach a nursing strand but the remainder of the curriculum will be controlled by life scientists or social scientists. In such a situation, how will the integration of theory and practice, so central to all these proposals for change, actually be accomplished?

Once again, in fact, there are striking parallels with developments in medicine, where the pre-clinical programme is increasingly defined and taught by non-clinical scientists rather than doctors, although the reasons are somewhat different.[8] There is a certain irony in the way in which professionalization in nursing has often been identified with the weakening of medical control. It is, however, conceivable that the attempt to imitate medical models of career structures and educational organization in an environment which nurses do not control may actually further reduce the ability of nursing to determine its own fate.

It is this tendency to ignore environmental factors that fatally flaws all three sets of proposals. Most crucially, all three deal evasively with the critical issues of demography and cost. These, though, are the points which are of critical concern to anyone involved in planning or managing health care.

The one brute demographic fact on which everyone is agreed is that the traditional pool of recruitment for nursing — girls with 5 'O' Levels or 2 'A' Levels — will contract until the mid 1990s and will not recover to the levels of the 1970s and 1980s in the present century. On current trends, nursing would need to recruit almost half of this population by 1995 in competition with higher education, other health and welfare occupations, teaching and the wider employment opportunities for women resulting from the weakening of sex discrimination. Just to state this is to recognize its implausibility. It is, in essence, the same problem as the occupation faced in the 1930s, partly as a result of its success in squeezing out the handywoman class.

There is no obvious solution. The professionalizers appear to favour moves to strengthen the competitive position of nursing by increasing the attractiveness of its training, working conditions and salaries. The managers seem to prefer the idea of dilution, looking for nursing tasks that could be performed by less expensive and more readily available labour. Both also at least acknowledge the option of trying to widen the pool of recruitment by introducing routes into the occupation which are less dependent on formal educational credentials and less bound to recruits from a narrow age bracket and a particular gender.

The professional solution embodied in the ENB, RCN and UKCC reports and associated documents appears, at first sight, to have substantial cost and staffing implications. It would greatly reduce the labour input from students on hospital wards and require considerable extra investment in educational facilities. The economic advice commissioned by these interests, however, suggests that the net costs could be greatly reduced by paying students at the level of grants prevailing in higher education rather than a competitive wage and by reducing wastage during training, thereby reducing the number of people that it is necessary to recruit in order to achieve a particular output. There would also be gains from a reduction in the amount of time spent by ward staff in teaching. These measures would save almost enough to cover the cost of additional auxiliary labour. Goodwin and Bosanquet (1986), for instance, estimate that the net cost of the RCN proposals would be about £32 million. The UKCC, assuming a higher labour input from students, was advised by Price Waterhouse accountants that its scheme could be introduced without additional expenditure.

But these estimates have been treated with scepticism by their policy audience. The assumptions about wastage, for example, are based on the experience of present-day degree programmes with a highly selected and motivated intake. It is not obvious that they can be generalized to a mass entry. Even if they can, the result may be only to defer wastage until after the completion of training when students cease to be sheltered from the demands of ward life. One advantage of the present system is that early wastage does not waste resources. Related to this is the view, expressed in private discussions at one of the accrediting bodies in higher education, that if nurses have a qualification with a more clearly defined academic value, this will actually make it easier for them to leave the occupation, the fear of the hospitals before the First World War.

Similarly, if students are to be paid grants at the prevailing levels in higher education, assuming a grant system continues to operate, the question must be raised about the competitiveness of nursing courses. Will students with a general motivation towards health and welfare work really be attracted in competition with other paramedical or social work programmes which may be less demanding in terms of their clinical commitments and lead to better paid and more flexible careers? Finally, managers are intrinsically suspicious of claims that reducing student presence on the ward will free more existing staff time for patient care. It is equally likely that more time will be consumed in supervising students with less well-developed practical skills or in managing the auxiliary labour.

The status of these auxiliaries is really the crucial question for the whole debate. The professionalizer's proposals, for instance, remain almost silent on this point, possibly because they regard the auxiliary role as negligible. The RCN aspires to a wholly qualified workforce, while the UKCC envisages 70 per cent of care being delivered by registered practitioners. Their main objective appears to be to draw a sharper line between registered nurses and auxiliaries or helpers. This seems to be an important element in the desire to eliminate the SEN grade, for example.

It is the moment at which the limitations of a 'nurse-centric' approach become clear. As the Institute of Health Service Management observes in its comments on Project 2000:

> Nurses sometimes perform duties simply because they happen to be on the spot. The various contributions and roles of other groups such as clerical or ancillary staff need to be taken into account in building up a complete picture of the staffing functions in an environment such as a hospital ward. (Institute of Health Service Management 1987)

The management interests are much further advanced in such discussions than the professionalizers.[9]

For some reason, however, they have been reluctant to show their hand too publicly. The NHS Training Authority report, *Support Workers to Nurses, Midwives and Health Visitors: The Role, Selection and Training Issues*, ceased to be available shortly after its publication in March 1987. Its view of this grade is radically at odds with that of the nursing reports. The NHSTA envisages support workers having a clear and direct responsibility for patient care, including preparing for and assisting in clinical procedures, making and recording observations and performing rehabilitation tasks. In contrast to present day auxiliaries, they would have specific training for this task which would form part of a modular pattern of education extending right across the service. Part of the entry might come from unqualified school leavers on YTS schemes, part from mature men and women with limited past educational opportunities. An appropriate accumulation of credits would qualify support workers for entry to nurse training.

The NHSTA proposals reflect wider political and educational enthusiasms for 'ladders and bridges', credit accumulation schemes that provide flexible educational opportunities in adult life. They are inspired by the same ideals as the setting up of the National Council for Vocational Qualifications which has been charged with producing an integrated system of credentials for vocational training across the entire labour market. All certificates, diplomas, etc. will be graded relative to one another and pathways identified that will permit people with few formal qualifications to identify an appropriate entry point and self-development track.

For nursing, of course, one consequence would be a blurring rather than a sharpening of grade boundaries. These proposals anticipate wards staffed with a more complex mixture of personnel. In effect the reduction in the availability of students with different skill levels depending on the stage of progress in their training would be made up by the introduction of auxiliaries with a variety of skill levels, at least some of whom might be en route to nurse registration themselves. Quite apart from the flexibility of such a labour force, from a managerial point of view, it might also make the auxiliaries' job more attractive. One of the disadvantages of the professional model of the support worker is that by moving the auxiliary closer to the ward cleaner or maid, the recruitment difficulties of nursing may be compounded by the reluctance of existing auxiliary staff to remain and of others to come forward for what they will see as downgraded work.

In considering the future, it may be instructive to recall the history of the SEN. As Abel-Smith (1960) stressed, much of the history of nursing regulation can be seen as a struggle over the control of a 'second portal', the existence of a skilled grade of hospital worker assisting the registered nurse. Throughout the occupation's history a professionalist segment has sought to squeeze out the handywoman class from the care of the sick. In the metaphor of Chapter 1, they have sought to gentrify the plot of work owned by the occupation. The result has been a chronic problem of recruitment, which has occasionally been concealed by demographic bulges. There simply are not enough well-educated young women to whom the work is attractive to give all the personal care that the sick require. Even if there were, it is not clear that this would be an efficient use of the human resources available to our society. When recruitment last ran into a crisis in the late 1930s, the professionalizers' demands for an expansion of the registered nurse workforce were ignored by the interest of the hospitals and, after the outbreak of war, the ministry in the provision of adequate care at reasonable cost. With great reluctance, nursing was obliged to accept the SEN in order to have some influence over the growth of assistant nurses and to regulate their competition with SRN grades. The reports of the 1980s reopen this struggle but it is by no means obvious that the outcome is likely to be any different.[10] As Baly observes:

> The purists may fulminate, and legislation may change the legal position of the nurse, but whether she is village nurse, ordinary probationer, or enrolled nurse, it seems that nursing will always need some kind of two-tier system. Either there are not enough wholly trained people to undertake all the tasks, or there is not enough money to pay for them, or maybe all tasks do not require highly trained nurses, merely highly trained supervision. (Baly 1987: 56)

Views of the future

In this concluding chapter, as so often in the book, we have found ourselves ranging over a wide terrain at great speed. That, in itself, is one token of the sheer complexity of any attempt to understand this varied and fragmented occupation. Even at this length, it has been necessary to neglect important issues like the debate over the future organization of primary care and the place of nursing within it. In a sense we have ourselves reproduced the ideological dominance of general nursing. And yet this may not be entirely indefensible given that it is likely that the concerns of general nursing will have the greatest influence on the future shape of the occupation and that other segments will be remade to fit with them. For the last hundred years the general hospital has been the key battleground for the various forces arrayed in the division of labour in health care. There seems no reason why this should change now.

What we do hope to have shown in this book, however, is that the shape of nursing cannot be entirely understood from within. Nursing is one interest in a division of labour whose boundaries are in a constant state of flux. Indeed this is part of its very fascination for students of occupations. Located as it is between a powerful profession jealous of its own freedom and prestige and the pervasive social concern of the economical management of deviance, the state of nursing is an early indicator of more profound social changes. The nursing process, for instance, predates many of the political changes which have legitimated its reconstruction of nurse/patient relationships on the model of private practice.

We do not have a crystal ball but there are clearly a number of options for the future of nursing. Purely on demographic grounds the status quo is not one of them. Melia (1987) sketches out an appealing model in her suggestion of a reconstruction along craft principles. Rather than emphasizing the elitism of a profession, nurses should look to the autonomy of the craft worker, performing a trade with considerable skill, judgement, and self-direction, with the support of journeymen, apprentices and labourers. An alternative vision might draw more directly on US experience, emphasizing the scope for diluting the medical profession with specialized nurses. Clinical specialists might take over the routine management of large groups of patients, especially in obstetrics, paediatrics, geriatrics and psychiatry. In the long term, we might see renewed fission and some of these groups splitting off to form new paramedical specialties like speech therapy, physiotherapy and the rest. On this scenario, it may be that the ward sister ceases to become the core nursing role and is translated into the first level of general management.

But, if we ask who will be standing beside the patient's bed in hospital providing the direct hands-on routine care in the year 2000, it is difficult to resist the conclusion that it will still be the handywoman class in the new guise of support workers. Indeed, they are also likely to dominate non-hospital, non-family care. The great challenge for the official occupation of nursing is to find a way of doing justice to those true heirs to the title. Professional ambitions must be reconciled with economic realities. No elitist programme of nursing reform has yet been allowed to succeed. Would an alternative based on open entry and continuing opportunity have more prospects of serving both the occupation and its public?

Notes

Chapter 1 Nurses and Servants

1. Larson's approach is very similar to that of most economists who define a profession as a type of legally protected monopoly in the supply of certain services (e.g. Forgotson and Cook 1967, Hodgson 1977, Smith *et al.* 1979, cf. Dingwall and Fenn 1987, Gray 1987).
2. Unfortunately Reverby's (1987) account of the development of American nursing only became available in the UK as this book was being completed. There are, however, many striking parallels in the development of nursing in the two countries, in this early period and later, which reflect the constraints on caring work in a market society. In each case, the historical record has also been substantially mythologized to obscure the contribution of ordinary working-class women to that work.

Chapter 2 The Revolution in Nursing

1. Army medicine, in both Britain and France, was something of an exception to the stagnation of technical development during the eighteenth century, partly at least because it was the one sector where doctors were not beholden to their patients and had the authority to impose treatments (Jewson 1974: 384–5).
2. Louisa Twining was a daughter of the family of tea merchants, who formed the Workhouse Visiting Society in 1858, 'to promote the moral and spiritual improvement of workhouse inmates'. This had 140 members visiting 12 London workhouses in 1860 and several provincial branches (Abel-Smith 1960: 38). It provided a network of contacts out of which grew a small number of other associations for the assistance of workhouse children, the support of unmarried mothers and the rehabilitation of prostitutes (Crowther 1981: 68–70).

Chapter 3 The New Model Nurse

1. Octavia Hill (1838–1912) was a prominent member of the movement to reform housing conditions for the poor both by the provision of

accommodation and by active management of tenants' lives to encourage habits of thrift, which would enable them to pay the rent, and sobriety, which would lead the property to be treated with respect. She was one of the founders of the Charity Organisation Society, which we discuss on pp.177–8.

2. The potential tribulations of the governess are vividly depicted in several of the novels of the Bronte sisters who came from precisely this impoverished stratum of the middle class and had experienced work of this kind. See especially Anne's *Agnes Grey* (1847) and Charlotte's *Jane Eyre* (1847) and *Shirley* (1849).

Chapter 4 Making the Myths

1. Maggs (1987: 187) quotes a figure of 'nearly £4,000 net' as the London Hospital's profit for hiring out its staff. Abel-Smith (1960: 51–8) gives £3,957 as the gross income from this source of those London hospitals reporting to *Burdett's Annual* in 1901. The London Hospital earned £4,000 gross a year in this manner by 1905, leaving £1,700 as the net profit.

Chapter 5 The Search for Unity

1. Maggs's figures show an increase from £97 to £156 for nursing salary costs at 1898 rates on the assumption that probationers were unpaid and self-financed, as the registrationists proposed. If we assume that women would not have come forward in sufficient numbers on this basis and probationers continued to be paid the prevailing rates, the actual rise would be to £199, i.e. the extra costs of trained staff plus the wages paid to probationers.
2. See the discussion of the clashes between the LGB and the CMB on pp.160–1.
3. Overall, trade union membership increased from 2,565,000 in 1910 to 8,347,000 in 1920 (McKibbon 1974: 240).
4. An employers' combine is a tame union set up by employers to prevent the growth of a genuinely independent union.
5. This was a union of staff working in the lunatic asylums. Its history is discussed in Chapter 7 (pp.129–30).
6. There was a good deal of cross membership between these latter organizations which was to become important in the eventual selection of members for the first Council.
7. For further information on these Committees, see Abel-Smith (1964: 290–4, 307–11).
8. The register of mental nurses contained a further subdivision of nurses for the mentally handicapped.

Chapter 6 The Nationalization of Nursing

1. The effects on midwifery are discussed in Chapter 8 (pp.168–9).

2. For extended accounts, see Honigsbaum (1979), Klein (1983), Pater (1983) and Webster (1988).
3. Full accounts of the debate around this legislation can be found in White (1982, 1985) and Abel-Smith (1960: 215–27).

Chapter 7 Mental Disorder and Mental Handicap

1. The significance of these concerns will be examined further in Chapter 9 in relation to the development of health visiting.
2. The Board of Control was established under the Mental Deficiency Act (1913) to take over the powers of the Lunacy Commissioners, who had supervised lunacy institutions since 1845. The Board of Control exercised responsibility for mental disorder and mental deficiency. In 1948 the board was absorbed into the NHS, and in 1959 it was abolished.

Chapter 8 Midwifery

1. Abel-Smith (1960) suggests that these were mostly established by doctors as an adjunct to their private practice or by retired nurses as a profitable investment. He accepts the contemporary criticism of their standards of care, which he attributes to their commercial orientation. But even large voluntary hospitals were under considerable financial stress during the inter-war period (Eckstein 1958: 44–53). It would be interesting to know the extent to which nursing homes functioned as an alternative to the pre-war nurses' co-operatives as a way of organizing private work. Were they a successor under different market conditions? It is also important to recognize that much of the criticism comes from official nursing interests. Were these homes actually being run by competent people who had been prevented from registering and were subsequently the victims of black propaganda from an occupation which was trying to establish what would now be called a 'market shelter', a privileged protection from competition? Sources like the Report of the Parliamentary Select Committee on Nursing Homes (HMSO 1926) contain enough evidence to accept that abuse did occur, but it seems implausible to suppose that the sector would have grown so rapidly if low standards were characteristic.
2. Many small rural infirmaries remained relatively unaffected by these developments and, of course, the sector as a whole still had the dominant role in the care of chronic or incurable patients. Even in large urban areas, this group continued to be treated under the local authorities' powers of poor relief and excluded from the improvements effected by the use of public health powers in the acute services. Excluding London, 42 per cent of public beds in urban areas in 1938 were still classified as Poor Law provision, rising to 77 per cent in the counties (Crowther 1986: 74).
3. It is a criminal offence for anyone other than a doctor or a registered midwife or a student in training for either occupation to deliver a baby.

Emergency service personnel or others who deliver a baby in exceptional circumstances are protected from prosecution only by the health authorities' discretion not to bring proceedings if they do not consider this to be in the public interest. It is not a criminal offence for an unqualified person to nurse the sick or, in some circumstances, to use the title 'nurse' as long as she does not pretend to be registered or enrolled.

4. Against this, Moscucci canvasses the possibility that some of these entries may be deliberately disingenuous, reflecting a tacit agreement between the woman and the doctor for the performance of an abortion. Although a criminal act, abortion does not seem to have been particularly stigmatized as a means of birth control for married middle-class women in the mid-nineteenth century.

5. Smith (1979: 13–14) argues that the rate for the 1830s is an underestimate because death certification was voluntary until 1874 and many deaths caused by childbirth were likely to have been classified under other causes such as peritonitis. Loudon (1986: 24–5) accepts this but points out that it would have been partly counterbalanced by a tendency to include 'associated deaths', i.e. deaths occurring within four to six weeks of giving birth from unrelated causes such as cholera outbreaks.

6. Sandelowski (1984) and Leavitt (1986) discuss how the demand for anaesthesia was also an important factor in the shift from midwives to doctors as birth attendants in the USA.

Chapter 9 District Nursing and Health Visiting

1. There has been a Rathbone at the heart of developments in district nursing ever since (Stocks 1960, Baly 1987: 131–2).

2. Mrs Robinson's antecedents are somewhat obscure. Baly (1986: 123) describes her as having worked at St Thomas's in the pre-Nightingale Fund era but later (1987: 6) refers to her as possibly trained at St John's. These statements are not necessarily inconsistent but the result is confusing.

3. Baly (1986: 124) identifies Rathbone's views with those of the COS in establishing the Liverpool scheme but this is plainly anachronistic: the Liverpool district nursing programme began in 1859, while the COS was not founded until 1869.

4. Salford had had a voluntary notification scheme since 1889 (Lane-Claypon 1920: 9).

Chapter 10 Professional Autonomy and Economic Constraints

1. 'Barbara' is Barbara Castle, Secretary of State for Employment and Productivity 1968–70.

2. The term 'bureaucracy' in social science does not have the pejorative implications that it often takes on in everyday usage. It was introduced by the German sociologist Max Weber (1947: 329–41) to describe a

particular type of organization which is common in modern societies. This is marked by an impersonal administration of formal rules, intended to guarantee equal treatment of everyone having dealings with the organization by minimizing the scope for employees to use their personal discretion. Equality tends to be valued over initiative. Most subsequent writing in social science has concentrated on what Weber called the 'monocratic' form of bureaucracy, where there is a single chain of command to a single head, but he also identified a 'collegial' form where there were parallel chains performing specialized functions whose joint consent is required for any decision. As he observed, such a system favours thoroughness in decision-making but is not conducive to 'rapid, clear decisions free of the necessity of compromise' (Weber 1947: 336).

3. The Merrison Committee (1975) examined the work of the General Medical Council and its report was reflected in the Medical Act 1978. This was consolidated with earlier legislation into a single comprehensive statute, the Medical Act 1983. Similar thinking is reflected in the Dentists Acts 1983 and 1984.

4. When Dingwall and McIntosh were completing the compilation of their book of readings on the sociology of nursing early in 1977, for example, the nursing process was still not identified as a distinctive social movement. Although several of the key American references are cited (Dingwall and McIntosh 1978: 164), they are seen as part of a more general and varied debate on the quality of care rather than as exemplifying a particular 'party line'.

5. Turner (1978) analyses the reports of a number of public inquiries into major accidents or disasters and contrasts their emphasis on individual failures with the evidence that organizational breakdowns show common patterns of system collapse. Unless organization designers learn to recognize and accommodate these, efforts to change individual behaviour are unlikely to be successful in preventing new catastrophes. An application of these ideas to the field of health and social services can be found in Dingwall (1986), which reviews inquiries into child abuse deaths. The same principles apply if one examines other failures, like an unsuccessful attempt to introduce a practice innovation.

6. The Hawthorne Effect takes its name from a series of experiments conducted during the 1930s in the Hawthorne plant of the Western Electric company in the USA. The object was to measure the effect of physical changes in the working environment on levels of productivity, but the researchers found that whatever they did productivity seemed to keep increasing. They eventually concluded that this was due to the sense of value which the workers derived from their participation in the experiments and the individual attention which they received while being interviewed by members of the research team (Roethlisberger and Dickson 1939).

7. The Oxfordshire Strategy for Health Visiting, for example, proposes that each health visitor will compile an annual community health profile, which will inevitably be determined by those statistics which

have already been defined as worth collecting. She will then 'select *her* priorities, set objectives and make an action plan'. Her priorities will be determined by professionally devised 'vulnerability indices' or 'health assessments', again based on the professionals' assumptions about what will be important to clients or what it is appropriate to deal with.

8. They seem to be a combination of the limitations of a medical training in bringing doctors up to the level of specialist skills necessary for advanced teaching and research in the life sciences and the inferior pay and conditions of pre-clinical employment which are uncompetitive with those offered to clinicians.

9. As this book was completed, for example, it appears that the RCN had only just realized that any movement towards a more elite definition of nursing was likely to have the result of reducing its membership base. Private discussions of the possibility of creating an associate class of membership for auxiliaries were tempered by the recognition that these workers were already being organized by health service unions. Given that the whole objective of change was to increase the social distance between nurses and auxiliaries, it seemed unlikely that the latter would flock to become second-class members of the RCN. Nevertheless, the 1988 RCN Conference was persuaded to support proposals that could lead to the recruitment of auxiliaries or 'helpers'.

10. The conflicting interpretations of the Secretary of State's qualified acceptance of Project 2000 in his address to the 1988 RCN Conference merely underline our point. The initial enthusiasm of the professionalizers was rapidly dispelled by the DHSS press briefings which stressed the importance of the helper grades as a channel of recruitment, in line with the NHSTA proposals and looked forward to a workforce containing a significantly smaller proportion of registered nurses than current in the 1980s.

References

Abel-Smith, B. (1960) *A History of the Nursing Profession*, London: Heinemann.

Abel-Smith, B. (1964) *The Hospitals 1800–1948: A Study in Social Administration in England and Wales*, London: Heinemann.

Abbott, A. (1986) 'Jurisdictional Conflicts: A New Approach to the Development of the Legal Profession', *American Bar Foundation Research Journal* 1986: 187–224.

Adams, F. (1969) 'From Association to Union: Professional Organisation of Asylum Attendants, 1869–1919', *British Journal of Sociology*, 20: 11–26.

Alaszewski, A. (1983) 'The Development of Policy for the Mentally Handicapped Since the Second World War', in J. Gabbay (ed.) *Oxford Review of Education* 'Special Issue: Mental Handicap and Education', 9: 227–32.

Allan, P. and Jolley, M. (1982) *Nursing, Midwifery and Health Visiting since 1900*, London: Faber.

Altschul, A.T. (1963) 'Trends in Psychiatric Nursing', in H. Freeman and J. Farndale (eds) *Trends in the Mental Health Services*, Oxford: Pergamon.

Andrews, C.T. (1975) *The First Cornish Hospital*, privately published, Truro.

Armstrong, D. (1983) *Political Anatomy of the Body: Medical Knowledge in Britain in the Twentieth Century*, Cambridge, UK: Cambridge University Press.

Aubert, V. and Messinger, S. (1958) 'The Criminal and the Sick', *Inquiry*, 1: 137–60.

Aveling, J.H. (1887) *The Chamberlens and the Midwifery Forceps*, London: J. & A. Churchill.

Baly, M. (1986) *Florence Nightingale and the Nursing Legacy*, London: Croom Helm.

Baly, M. (1987) *A History of the Queen's Institute: 100 Years 1887–1987*, London: Croom Helm.

Beardshaw, V. (1982) *Conscientious Objectors at Work: Mental Hospital Nurses: A Case Study*, London: Social Audit.

Becker, H.S. (1970) 'The Nature of a Profession', in H.S. Becker *Sociological Work*, Chicago: Aldine.

Behlmer, G.K. (1982) *Child Abuse and Moral Reform in England 1870–1908*, Stanford: Stanford University Press.

Bendall, E. and Raybould, E. (1969) *A History of the General Nursing Council for England and Wales 1919–1969*, London: H.K. Lewis.

Berger, P. and Luckmann, T. (1971) *The Social Construction of Reality*, Harmondsworth: Penguin.

Birchenall, P.D. (1982), 'Mental Handicap Nursing', in P. Allan and M. Jolley (eds) *Nursing, Midwifery and Health Visiting since 1900*, London: Faber.

Board of Control (1915–1938) *Annual Reports*, London: HMSO.

Board of Control (1922) *Lunacy Reform Conference, January 1922*, London: HMSO.

Board of Control (1924) *Report of the Departmental Committee appointed to inquire into the nursing service in county and borough mental hospitals*, London: HMSO.

Board of Control (1925) *The Nursing Service in Mental Hospitals, Conference, April 1925*, London: HMSO.

Board of Control (1930) *Mental Treatment, Conference, July 1930*, London: HMSO.

Bowman, G., Thompson, D., and Sutton, D. (1983) 'Nurses' Attitudes Towards the Nursing Process', *Journal of Advanced Nursing* 8: 125–9.

Brickman, J.P. (1983) 'Public Health, Midwives and Nurses 1880–1930', in E.C. Lagemann (ed.) *Nursing History: New Perspectives, New Possibilities*, New York: Teachers' College Press.

Brittain, V. (1978) *Testament of Youth*, London: Virago.

Brooking, J. (1986) 'Patient and Family Participation in Nursing Care: The Development of a Nursing Process Measuring Scale', Ph.D. thesis, King's College, University of London.

Budge, U.V. (1967) 'Psychiatric Nurse Training and its Implications for Patient Care', in H. Freeman and J. Farndale (eds) *New Aspects of the Mental Health Services*, Oxford: Pergamon.

Bullough, V.L. and Bullough, B. (1979) *The Care of the Sick: The Emergence of Modern Nursing*, London: Croom Helm.

Busfield, J. (1986) *Managing Madness*, London: Hutchinson.

Caplow, T.A. (1954) *The Sociology of Work*, Minneapolis: University of Minnesota Press.

Carpenter, M. (1977a) 'The New Managerialism and Professionalism in Nursing', in M. Stacey, M. Reid, C. Heath and R. Dingwall (eds) *Health and the Division of Labour*, London: Croom Helm.

Carpenter, M. (1977b) 'Managerialism and the Division of Labour in Nursing', in R. Dingwall and J. McIntosh (eds) *Readings in the Sociology of Nursing*, Edinburgh: Churchill Livingstone.

Carpenter, M. (1980) 'Asylum Nursing Before 1914: a Chapter on the History of Labour', in C. Davies (ed.) *Rewriting Nursing History*, London: Croom Helm.

Carpenter, M. (1982) 'The Labour Movement in the National Health

Service', in A.S. Sethi and S.J. Dimmock (eds) *Industrial Relations and Health Services*, London: Croom Helm.

Carpenter, M. (1985) *They Still Go Marching On: A Celebration of COHSE's First 75 Years*, London: Confederation of Health Service Employees.

Central Health Services Council (1968) *Psychiatric Nursing Today and Tomorrow*, London: HMSO.

Central Statistical Office (1987) *Annual Abstract of Statistics 1987*, London: HMSO.

Clark, P. (1979) 'Migration in England During the Late Seventeenth and Early Eighteenth Centuries', *Past and Present* 83: 57–90.

Cook, E.T. (1913) *The Life of Florence Nightingale*, 2 vols, London: Macmillan.

Cooper, D. (1971) *The Death of the Family*, Harmondsworth: Penguin.

Cooper, Lady Diana (1958) *The Rainbow Comes and Goes*, Reprinted London: Century Press, 1984.

Cope, D.E. (1981) *Organisation Development and Action in Hospitals*, Aldershot: Gower.

Cope, Z. (1958) *Florence Nightingale and the Doctors*, London: Museum Press.

Council for the Education and Training of Health Visitors (1977) *An Investigation into the Principles of Health Visiting*, London: CETHV.

Council for the Education and Training of Health Visitors (1980) *The Investigation Debate*, London: CETHV.

Council for the Education and Training of Health Visitors (1982) *Health Visiting: Principles in Practice*, London: CETHV.

Cowell, B. and Wainwright, D. (1981) *Behind the Blue Door: The History of the Royal College of Midwives 1881–1981*, London: Bailliere Tindall.

Crossman, R.H.S. (1977) *The Crossman Diaries: Vol.III*, London: Hamish Hamilton/Jonathan Cape.

Crowther, M.A. (1981) *The Workhouse System 1834–1929*, London: Batsford.

Crowther, M.A. (1986) 'Medicine and the End of the Poor Law', *Bulletin of the Society for the Social History of Medicine*, 38: 74–6.

Davies, C. (1980) 'Making Sense of the Census', *Sociological Review*, 28: 581–609.

Davies, C. (1985) 'Policy in Nursing Education: Plus ca change', *Proceedings of the 19th Annual Study Day of the Warnig Studies Association*, Edinburgh: University of Edinburgh.

Davies, C. (1988) 'The Health Visitor as Mother's Friend: A Woman's Place in Public Health 1900–1914', *Social History of Medicine*, 1: 39–60.

Davin, A. (1978) 'Imperialism and Motherhood', *History Workshop* 5: 9–65.

De la Cuesta, C. (1983) 'The Nursing Process: From Development to Implementation', *Journal of Advanced Nursing* 8: 365–71.

Dean, M. and Bolton, G. (1980) 'The Administration of Poverty and the Development of Nursing Practice in 19th Century England', in C.

Davies (ed.) *Rewriting Nursing History*, London: Croom Helm.

DHSS (1971) *Better Services for the Mentally Handicapped*, Cmnd. 4683, London: HMSO.

DHSS (1975) *Better Services for the Mentally Ill*, Cmnd. 6233, London: HMSO.

DHSS (1976–81) *Development Team for the Mentally Handicapped: Reports*, London: DHSS.

DHSS (1980) *Organisational and Management Problems of Mental Illness Hospitals. Report of a Working Group* (Chairman, T.E. Nodder), London: DHSS.

DHSS (1983) *NHS Management Inquiry DA (83) 38* (Chairman Mr. R. Griffiths), London: DHSS.

DHSS/OPCS/Welsh Office (1986) *Hospital In-Patient Enquiry: Maternity Tables 1977–81*, Series MB4 No. 19, London: HMSO.

DHSS/Scottish Home and Health Department/Welsh Office (1970) *Report of the Working Party on Management Structure in the Local Authority Nursing Services* (Chairman, E.L. Mayston), London: HMSO.

DHSS/Welsh Office/CHSC (1968) *Psychiatric Nursing Today and Tomorrow*, London: HMSO.

Dickson, N. (1987), 'Quality Assurance: Do you measure up?', *Nursing Times* 83: 25–8.

Digby, A. (1978) *Pauper Palaces*, London: Routledge & Kegan Paul.

Digby, A. (1985) *Madness, Morality and Medicine: A Study of the York Retreat 1796–1914*, Cambridge, UK: Cambridge University Press.

Dingwall, R. (1974) 'Some Sociological Aspects of Nursing Research', *Sociological Review* 22: 45–55.

Dingwall, R. (1977a) *Aspects of Illness*, London: Martin Robertson.

Dingwall, R. (1977b) 'Collectivism, Regionalism and Feminism: Health Visiting and British Social Policy 1850–1975', *Journal of Social Policy* 6: 291–315.

Dingwall, R. (1979) 'The Place of Men in Nursing', in M. Colledge and D. Jones (eds) *Readings in Nursing*, Edinburgh: Churchill Livingstone.

Dingwall, R. (1983a) 'Introduction', in R. Dingwall and P. Lewis (eds) *The Sociology of the Professions: Lawyers, Doctors and Others*, London: Macmillan.

Dingwall, R. (1983b) 'In the Beginning Was the Work . . . Reflections on the Genesis of Occupations', *Sociological Review* 31: 605–24.

Dingwall, R. (1986) 'The Jasmine Beckford Affair', *Modern Law Review* 49: 489–507.

Dingwall, R. and Eekelaar, J.M. (1988) 'Families and the State: An Historical Perspective on the Public Regulation of Private Conduct', *Law and Policy*, forthcoming.

Dingwall, R. and Fenn, P. (1987) 'A Respectable Profession: Sociological and Economic Perspectives on the Regulation of Professional Services', *International Review of Law and Economics* 7: 51–64.

Dingwall, R., Eekelaar, J.M. and Murray, T. (1983) *The Protection of Children: State Intervention and Family Life*, Oxford: Basil Blackwell.

Dingwall, R., Eekelaar, J.M. and Murray, T. (1984) 'Childhood as a Social Problem: A Survey of the History of Legal Regulation', *Journal*

239

References

of Law and Society, 11: 207–32.

Dingwall, R. and McIntosh, J. (eds) (1978) Readings in the Sociology of Nursing, Edinburgh: Churchill Livingstone.

Doerner, K. (1981) Madness and the Bourgeoisie. A Social History of Insanity and Psychiatry, Oxford: Basil Blackwell.

Donajgrodzki, A.P. (1977) Social Control in Nineteenth Century Britain, London: Croom Helm.

Donnison, J. (1977) Midwives and Medical Men: A History of Inter-Professional Rivalries and Women's Rights, London: Heinemann.

Donzelot, J. (1980) The Policing of Families, London: Hutchinson.

Dowling, W.C. (1963) 'The Ladies' Sanitary Association and the Origin of the Health Visiting Service', MA dissertation, London School of Economics.

Drake, B. (1920) Women in Trade Unions (reprinted 1984), London: Virago.

Dwork, D. (1986) War is Good for Babies and Other Young Children: A History of the Infant and Child Welfare Movement in England 1898–1918, London: Tavistock.

Dyehouse, C. (1978) 'Working Class Mothers and Infant Mortality in England 1895–1914', Journal of Social History 12: 248–69.

Eckstein, H. (1958) The English Health Service: Its Origins, Structure and Achievements, Cambridge, Mass.: Harvard University Press.

English National Board for Nursing, Midwifery and Health Visiting (1985) Professional Education/Training Courses: Consultation Paper, London: ENB.

Evans, K. (1975), The Development and Structure of the English Educational System, London: Athlone Press.

Everest, R. (1982) 'Mental Illness Nursing', in P. Allan and M. Jolley (eds) Nursing, Midwifery and Health Visiting since 1900, London: Faber.

Fears, M. (1977) 'Therapeutic Optimism and the Treatment of the Insane', in R. Dingwall, C. Heath, M. Reid and M. Stacey (eds) Health Care and Health Knowledge, London: Croom Helm.

Fears, M. (1978) 'The Moral Treatment of Insanity: A Study in the Social Construction of Human Nature', unpublished Ph.D. Thesis, University of Edinburgh.

Ferguson, T.S. (1958) Scottish Social Welfare 1864–1914, Edinburgh: E. & S. Livingstone.

Ferguson, S. and Fitzgerald, H. (1954) Studies in the Social Services, London: HMSO/Longmans Green.

Fido, J. (1977) 'The Charity Organisation Society and Social Casework in London 1869–1900', in A.P. Donajgrodzki (ed.) Social Control in Nineteenth Century Britain, London: Croom Helm.

Fitton, F. and Acheson, H.W.K. (1979) The Doctor–Patient Relationship in General Practice, London: HMSO.

Forgotson, E.H. and Cook, J.L. (1967) 'Innovations and Experiments in Uses of Health Manpower – The Effect of Licensure Laws', Law and Contemporary Problems 31: 731–50.

Foucault, M. (1965) Madness and Civilisation, London: Tavistock.

240

Foucault, M. (1973) *The Birth of the Clinic*, London: Tavistock.

Foucault, M. (1979) *Discipline and Punish: The Birth of the Prison*, New York: Vintage Books.

Freidson, E. (1970a) *Profession of Medicine*, New York: Dodd, Mead.

Freidson, E. (1970b) *Professional Dominance: The Social Structure of Medical Care*, New York: Atherton.

Freidson, E. (1978) 'The Official Construction of Work: An Essay on the Practical Epistemology of Occupations', paper presented at the Ninth World Congress of Sociology, Uppsala.

Freidson, E. (1983) 'The Theory of Professions: State of the Art', in R. Dingwall and P. Lewis (eds) *The Sociology of the Professions: Lawyers, Doctors and Others*, London: Macmillan.

Freidson, E. (1986) *Professional Powers: A Study of the Institutionalization of Formal Knowledge*, Chicago: University of Chicago Press.

Gabbay, J. (ed.) (1983) 'Special Issue: Mental Handicap and Education', *Oxford Review of Education* 9, No. 3.

Gamarnikow, E. (1978) 'Sexual Division of Labour: The Case of Nursing', in A. Kuhn and A. Wolpe (eds) *Feminism and Materialism: Women and Modes of Production*, London: Routledge & Kegan Paul.

Garland, D. (1985) *Punishment and Welfare: A History of Penal Strategies*, Aldershot: Gower.

Gilbert, B.B. (1966) *The Evolution of National Insurance in Great Britain: The Origins of the Welfare State*, London: Michael Joseph.

Gilbert, B.B. (1970) *British Social Policy 1914–1939*, London: Batsford.

Goffman, E. (1969) 'The Insanity of Place', *Psychiatry* 32: 357–87.

Goodwin, L. and Bosanquet, N. (1986) *Nurses and Higher Education: The Costs of Change*, York: University of York, Centre for Health Economics.

Goody, J.R. (1958) *The Developmental Cycle in Domestic Groups*, Cambridge, UK: Cambridge University Press.

Gray, A. (1987) *The Economics of Nursing: A Literature Review*, Coventry: University of Warwick, Nursing Policy Studies Centre.

Greenwood, E. (1957) 'The Attributes of a Profession', *Social Work* 2: 44–55.

Gubrium, J. (1975) *Living and Dying at Murray Manor*, New York: St Martin's Press.

Gubrium, J. (1980) 'Doing Care Plans in Patient Conferences', *Social Science and Medicine*, 14A: 659–67.

Gubrium, J. and Buckholdt, D. (1982) *Describing Care: Image and Practice in Rehabilitation*, Cambridge, Mass.: Oelgeschlager, Gunn and Hain.

Hair, P.E.H. (1982) 'Children in Society 1850–1980', in T. Barker and M. Drake (eds) *Population and Society in Britain 1850–1980* London: Batsford.

Harrison, B. (1967) 'Religion and Recreation in Nineteenth Century England', *Past and Present* 38: 108–19.

Hawker, R. (1985) 'A Day in the Life of a Patient', *Nursing Times* 12 June, 43–4.

References

Hawker, R. (1987) 'For the Good of the Patient?', in C. Maggs (ed.) *Nursing History: The State of the Art*, London: Croom Helm.

Hayward, J. (1986) *Report of the Nursing Process Evaluation Working Group*, London: King's College, University of London, Nursing Education Research Unit.

Hector, W. (1973) *The Life of Mrs. Bedford Fenwick*, London: Royal College of Nursing.

Henriques, U.R.Q. (1979) *Before the Welfare State: Social Administration in Early Industrial Britain*, London: Longman.

HMSO (1904) *Report from the Select Committee on Registration of Nurses, House of Commons*, London: HMSO.

HMSO (1905) *Report from the Select Committee on Registration of Nurses, House of Commons*, London: HMSO.

HMSO (1926) *Report from the Select Committee on Nursing Homes (Registration), House of Commons*, London: HMSO.

HMSO (1937) *Report on an Investigation into Maternal Mortality*, Cmd.5422, London: HMSO.

HMSO (1943) *Report of the Midwives Salaries Committee* (Chairman, Lord Rushcliffe) Cmd.6460, London: HMSO.

HMSO (1945) *Report by Sir Walter Monckton, K.C.M.G., K.C.V.O., M.C., K.C. on the circumstances which led to the boarding-out of Denis and Terence O'Neill at Bank Farm, Minsterly and the steps taken to supervise their welfare*, Cmd.6636, London: HMSO.

HMSO (1946) *Report of the Care of Children Committee* (Chairman, Dame Myra Curtis), Cmd.6922, London: HMSO.

HMSO (1956) *Report of the Committee of Enquiry into the Cost of the National Health Service* (Chairman, C.W. Guillebaud), Cmd.9663, London: HMSO.

HMSO (1968a) *Report of the Royal Commission on Medical Education* (Chairman, Lord Todd), Cmd.3569, London: HMSO.

HMSO (1968b) *Report of the Committee on Local Authority and Allied Personal Social Services* (Chairman, Lord Seebohm), Cmd.3703, London: HMSO.

HMSO (1972) *Report of the Committee on Nursing* (Chairman, Lord Briggs), Cmd.5115, London: HMSO.

HMSO (1975) *Report of the Committee of Enquiry into The Regulation of the Medical Profession* (Chairman, Sir Alec Merrison), Cmd.6018, London: HMSO.

HMSO (1976) *Report of the Committee on Child Health Services: Fit for the Future* (Chairman, Professor D. Court) 2 vols, Cmd.6684 and 6684–I, London: HMSO.

HMSO (1978) *Report of the Committee of Enquiry into the Education of Handicapped Children and Young People: Special Educational Needs* (Chairman, M. Warnock), Cmd. 7212, London: HMSO.

HMSO (1979) *Report of the Committee of Enquiry into Mental Handicap Nursing and Care* (Chairman, P. Jay) Cmd. 7468, London: HMSO.

Hodgkinson, R. (1967) *The Origins of the National Health Service*, London: Wellcome Historical Medical Library.

Hodgson, E.L. (1977) 'Restrictions on Unorthodox Health Treatment in

California: A Legal and Economic Analysis', *UCLA Law Review* 24: 647–6.

Honigsbaum, F. (1979) *The Division in British Medicine*, London: Kogan Page.

Hopkins, E. (1982) 'Working Hours and Conditions during the Industrial Revolution: A Re-appraisal', *Economic History Review* 35: 52–66.

Horobin, G.W. (1983) 'Professional Mystery: The Maintenance of Charisma in General Medical Practice', in R. Dingwall and P. Lewis (eds) *The Sociology of the Professions: Lawyers, Doctors and Others*, London: Macmillan.

Hughes, E.C. (1971) *The Sociological Eye*, Chicago: Aldine.

Hunter, R. and MacAlpine, I. (1974) *Psychiatry for the Poor*, London: Dawson.

Hutt, C.W. (1921) *Hygiene for Health Visitors, School Nurses and Social Workers*, London: Methuen.

Institute of Health Service Management (1987) 'Comments on Project 2000', London: Institute of Health Service Management.

Isaacs, S. (1941) *Cambridge Evacuation Survey*, London: Methuen.

Jaehnig, W. (1979) *A Family Service for the Mentally Handicapped*, London: Fabian Society.

Jewson, N.D. (1974) 'Medical Knowledge and the Patronage System in 18th Century England', *Sociology* 8: 369–85.

Jewson, N.D. (1976) 'The Disappearance of the Sick-Man from Medical Cosmology 1770–1870', *Sociology* 10: 225–44.

Johnson, T.J. (1972) *Professions and Power*, London: Macmillan.

Johnson, T.J. (1977) 'The Professions in the Class Structure', in R. Scase (ed.) *Industrial Society: Class, Cleavage and Control*, London: Allen & Unwin.

Johnson, T.J. (1982) 'The State and the Professions: Peculiarities of the British', in A. Giddens and G. Mackenzie, *Social Class and the Division of Labour: Essays in Honour of Ilya Neustadt*, Cambridge, UK: Cambridge University Press.

Jones, K. (1960) *Mental Health and Social Policy 1945–1959*, London: Routledge & Kegan Paul.

Keown, I.J. (1988) *Abortion, Doctors and the Law*, Cambridge, UK: Cambridge University Press.

Klein, R. (1983) *The Politics of the National Health Service*, London: Longman.

Lambert, W.R. (1975) 'Drink and Work-Discipline in Industrial South Wales c. 1800–1870', *Welsh Historical Review* 7: 289–306.

The *Lancet* (1932) *The Lancet Commission on Nursing*, London: The *Lancet*.

Lane-Claypon, J.E. (1920) *The Child Welfare Movement*, London: G. Bell and Sons.

Langton, B.M. (1963) 'Early Health Visiting', *Nursing Times* 4 October, 1247–8.

Larson, M.S. (1977) *The Rise of Professionalism: A Sociological Analysis*, Berkeley: University of California Press.

References

Laslett, P. (1983) *The World We Have Lost — Further Explored*, London: Methuen.

Leavitt, J.W. (1986) *Brought to Bed: Child-Bearing in America 1750–1950*, New York: Oxford University Press.

Lewis, J. (1980) *The Politics of Motherhood*, London: Croom Helm.

Local Government Board (1914–15) *Maternal Mortality in Relation to Childbirth: Supplement to the 44th Annual Report*, London: HMSO.

Local Government Board (1918) *Circular: Maternity and Child Welfare (M. & C.W. 4)*, London: Local Government Board.

Lomax, M. (1921) *The Experiences of an Asylum Doctor*, London: George Allen & Unwin.

Lonsdale, M. (1880) 'The Crisis at Guy's Hospital' *The Nineteenth Century* 40: 677–84.

Loudon, I.L., (1986) 'Deaths in Childbed from the Eighteenth Century to 1935', *Medical History* 30: 1–41.

Loudon, I.L. (1987) *Medical Care and the General Practitioner 1750–1850*, Oxford: Clarendon Press.

Loudon, I.L. (forthcoming) *Death in Childbirth: An International Study of Obstetric Care and Maternal Mortality*, Oxford: Oxford University Press.

McCleary, G.F. (1935) *The Maternity and Child Welfare Movement*, London: P.S. King.

MacDonald, M. (1981) *Mystical Bedlam: Madness, Anxiety, and Healing in Seventeenth Century England*, Cambridge, UK: Cambridge University Press.

McEwan, M. (1957) *Health Visiting*, London: Faber and Faber.

Macfarlane, A. and Mugford, M. (1984) *Birth Counts: Statistics of Pregnancy and Childbirth*, 2 vols, London: HMSO 1984.

McGregor, O.R., Blom-Cooper, L., and Gibson, C. (1970) *Separated Spouses*. London: Duckworth.

McIntosh, J. (1985) 'District Nursing: A Case of Political Marginality', in R. White (ed.) *Political Issues in Nursing: Past, Present and Future*, Chichester: John Wiley and Sons.

McKeown, T.S. (1965) *Medicine in Modern Society*, London: Allen & Unwin.

McKibbon, R. (1974) *The Evolution of the Labour Party 1910–1924*, Oxford: Oxford University Press.

Maggs, C.J. (1981) 'The Register of Nurses in the Scottish Poor Law Service 1885–1919' *Nursing Times* 77: 129–32.

Maggs, C.J. (1983) *The Origins of General Nursing*, London: Croom Helm.

Maggs, C.J. (1986) 'Sarey Gamp's Daughters: The English Nurse in Fiction', paper presented to Nursing and Anthropology Workshop, Oxford, 26/27 April.

Maggs, C.J. (1987) 'Profit and Loss and the Hospital Nurse', in C.J. Maggs (ed.) *Nursing History: The State of the Art*, London: Croom Helm.

Manson, T. (1977) 'Management, the Professions and the Unions: A Social Analysis of Change in the National Health Service', in

M. Stacey, M. Reid, C. Heath and R. Dingwall (eds) *Health and the Division of Labour*, London: Croom Helm.

Martin, J.P. (1984) *Hospitals in Trouble*, Oxford: Basil Blackwell.

Medico-Psychological Association (1885–1964) *Handbook for Attendants on the Insane*, London: Bailliere.

Melia, K. (1984) 'Student Nurses' Construction of Occupational Socialisation', *Sociology of Health and Illness* 6, 132–51.

Melia, K. (1987) *Learning and Working: The Occupational Socialization of Nurses*, London: Tavistock.

Mellett, D. (1982) *The Prerogative of Asylumdom*, New York: Gowland.

Menzies, I.E.P. (1963) 'A Case Study in the Functioning of Social Systems as a Defence Against Anxiety: A Report on a Study of the Nursing Service of a General Hospital', *Human Relations* 13: 95–121.

Millerson, G. (1964) *The Qualifying Associations: A study in Professionalization*, London: Routledge & Kegan Paul.

Ministry of Health (1919) *Circular: The Training of Health Visitors, Especially for Maternity and Child Welfare Work (M. & C.W. 10)*, London: Ministry of Health.

Ministry of Health (1949) *Report of the Working Party on Midwives*, London: HMSO.

Ministry of Health (1959) *Report of the Maternity Services Committee* (Chairman Lord Cranbrook), London: HMSO.

Ministry of Health and Board of Education (1939) *Interim Report of the Interdepartmental Committee on Nursing Services* (Chairman, The Earl of Athlone), London: HMSO.

Ministry of Health, Department of Health for Scotland, and Department of Education (1956) *An Inquiry into Health Visiting: Report of the Working Party* (Chairman, Sir Wilson Jameson), London: HMSO.

Ministry of Health and Ministry of Education (1945) Nursing Services Inter-Departmental Committee, *Report of Sub-Committee on Mental Nursing and the Nursing of the Mentally Defective*, London: HMSO.

Ministry of Health and Scottish Home and Health Department (1966) *Report of the Committee on Senior Nursing Staff Structure* (Chairman, B. Salmon), London: HMSO.

Ministry of Health, Department of Health for Scotland, and Ministry of Labour and National Service (1947) *Report of the Working Party on the Recruitment and Training of Nurses* (Chairman, Sir Robert Wood), London: HMSO.

Morgan, K. (1979) *Consensus and Disunity*, Oxford: Clarendon Press.

Moscucci, O. (1984) 'The Science of Women: British Gynaecology 1849–1890', D. Phil. Thesis, University of Oxford.

National Association for Mental Health (1961) *Emerging Patterns of the Mental Health Services*, London: National Association for Mental Health.

National Board for Prices and Incomes (1968) *Pay of Nurses and Midwives in the NHS: Report Number 60*, Cmd.3585, London: HMSO.

Newman, G. (1906) *Infant Mortality: A Social Problem*, London: Methuen.

Nightingale, F. (1859) *Notes on Nursing: What it is and what it is not*, London: Harrison and Sons.

References

Nolan, P. (1986) 'Mental Nurse Training in the 1920s', *Bulletin of the History of the Nursing Group* Spring 1986: 15–23.

Oakley, A. (1984) *The Captured Womb: A History of the Medical Care of Pregnant Women*, Oxford: Basil Blackwell.

Packman, J. (1975) *The Child's Generation*, Oxford: Basil Blackwell.

Parsons, T. (1952) *The Social System*, London: Routledge & Kegan Paul.

Parton, C. (1981) 'Liberal Individualism and Infant Mortality: The Infant Welfare Movement in Huddersfield 1900–18', MA thesis, Huddersfield Polytechnic.

Pater, J.E. (1983) *The Making of the National Health Service*, London: King's Fund.

Pearson, A. (1983) *The Clinical Nursing Unit*, London: Heinemann.

Pelling, H. (1968) *A Short History of the Labour Party*, London: Macmillan.

Pembrey, S. (1980) *The Ward Sister: Key to Nursing*, London: Royal College of Nursing.

Peretz, E. (in press) 'Infant Welfare in Oxford City 1919–1939 in R. Whiting (ed.) *Cities and Their People*, Manchester: Manchester University Press.

Platt, E. (1939) *The Story of the Ranyard Mission*, London: Hodder & Stoughton.

Poor Law Board (1866) *Metropolitan Workhouse Infirmaries and Sick Wards: Report of Dr Edward Smith, House of Lords Papers* 1866 (372) xi.

Porter, , R. (1983) 'The Rage of Party: A Glorious Revolution in English Psychiatry?' *Medical History* 27, 35–50.

Pritchard, D.G. (1963) *Education and the Handicapped 1760–1960*, London: Routledge & Kegan Paul.

Pyne, R. (1981) *Professional Discipline in Nursing: Theory and Practice*, Oxford: Blackwell Scientific.

Quaife, G.R. (1979) *Wanton Wenches and Wayward Wives: Peasants and Illicit Sex in Early Seventeenth Century England*, London: Croom Helm.

Reid, D.A. (1976) 'The Decline of Saint Monday 1766–1876', *Past and Present* 71:76–101.

Reid, M. (1983) 'Review Essay: A Feminist Sociological Imagination? Reading Ann Oakley', *Sociology of Health and Illness* 5: 83–94.

Reverby, S.M. (1987) *Ordered to Care: The Dilemma of American Nursing 1850–1945*, Cambridge, UK: Cambridge University Press.

Rivett, G. (1986) *The Development of the London Hospital System 1823–1982*, London: King's Fund.

Robb, B. (ed.) (1967) *Sans Everything: A Case to Answer*, Edinburgh: Thomas Nelson.

Roberts, R. (1973) *The Classic Slum*, Harmondsworth: Penguin.

Roberts, S. (1979) *Order and Dispute*, Oxford: Martin Robertson.

Robinson, J. and Strong, P.M. (1987) *Professional Nursing Advice After Griffiths: An Interim Report*. Coventry: University of Warwick, Nursing Policy Studies Centre.

Robson, P. (1983) 'Health Visiting: A Brief History', *Radical Health Visitors' Newsletter* 4.

Robson, P. (1986) 'The Development of Health Visiting in North-East England: A Case Study in Social Policy', in A. While (ed.) *Research in Preventative Community Nursing Care*, Chichester: John Wiley and Sons.

Roethlisberger, F.J. and Dickson, W.J. (1939) *Management and the Worker*, Cambridge, Mass.: Harvard University Press.

Rose, L. (1986) *Massacre of the Innocents: Infanticide in Great Britain 1800–1939*, London: Routledge & Kegan Paul.

Rosenberg, C.E. (in press) *The Care of Strangers: The Rise of America's Hospital System*, New York: Basic Books.

Roth, J. (1974) 'Professionalism: The Sociologist's Decoy', *Sociology of Work and Occupations* 1: 6–23.

Rothman, D. (1971) *The Discovery of the Asylum*, Boston: Little, Brown.

Royal College of Nursing (1948) *Memorandum on the Report of the Working Party on the Recruitment and Training of Nurses*, London: RCN.

Royal College of Nursing (1964) *A Reform of Nursing Education* (Chairman: Sir Anthony Platt), London: Royal College of Nursing.

Royal College of Nursing, Commission on Nursing Education (1985) *The Education of Nurses: A New Dispensation* (Judge Report). London: RCN.

Royal College of Obstetricians and Gynaecologists/Population Investigation Committee (1948) *Maternity in Great Britain: A Survey of Social and Economic Aspects of Pregnancy and Childbirth*, Oxford: Oxford University Press.

Runciman, S. (1983) *The Ward Sister at Work*, Edinburgh: Churchill Livingstone.

Russell, R. (1984) 'Mental Physicians and Their Patients', Ph. D. dissertation, University of Sheffield.

Ryan, J. with Thomas, K. (1980) *The Politics of Mental Handicap*, Harmondsworth: Penguin.

Sandelowski, M. (1984) *Pain, Pleasure and American Childbirth: From the Twilight Sleep to the Read Method 1914–1960*, Westport, Conn.: Greenwood Press.

Santos, E.V. and Stainbrook, E. (1949) 'A History of Psychiatric Nursing in the 19th Century', *Journal of the History of Medicine* 4: 48–74.

Scheff, T.J. (1963) 'Decision Rules, Types of Error and Their Consequences in Medical Diagnosis', *Behavioural Science* 8: 97–107.

Scull, A. (1979) *Museums of Madness: The Social Organisation of Insanity in 19th Century England*, London: Allen Lane.

Scull, A. (ed.) (1981) *Madhouses, Mad-Doctors and Madmen*, London: Athlone.

Seymer, L.R. (1954) *A General History of Nursing*, London: Faber and Faber.

Sharkey, S. (1880) 'Doctors and Nurses', *The Nineteenth Century* 40: 1097–1104.

Shryock, R. (1979) *The Development of Modern Medicine*, Madison: University of Wisconsin Press.

References

Silverman, D. (1987) *Communication and Medical Practice*, London: Sage.

Simnett, A. (1986) 'The Pursuit of Respectability: Women and the Nursing Profession', in R. White (ed.) *Political Issues in Nursing: Past, Present and Future Vol. 2*, Chichester: John Wiley and Sons.

Simon, S.D. (1938) *A Century of City Government: Manchester 1838–1938*, London: Allen & Unwin.

Smail, R. and Gray, A. (1982) *Nurses' Pay in the NHS*, Aberdeen: University of Aberdeen, Health Economics Research Unit.

Smith, F.B. (1979) *The People's Health 1830–1910*, London: Croom Helm.

Smith, F.B. (1982) *Florence Nightingale: Reputation and Power*, London: Croom Helm.

Smith, K.R., Miller, M. and Golladay, F. (1972) 'An Analysis of the Optimal Use of Inputs in the Production of Medical Services', *Journal of Human Resources* 7: 208–25.

South, J. (1857) *Facts relating to Hospital Nurses*, London.

Stedman Jones, G. (1971) *Outcast London: A Study in the Relationship Between Classes in Victorian Society*, Oxford: Clarendon Press.

Steele, Dr (1874) 'Report on the Nursing Arrangements of the London Hospitals', *British Medical Journal*, 285.

Stevens, R. (1966) *Medical Practice in Modern England: The Impact of Specialization and State Medicine*, New Haven: Yale University Press.

Stevenson, J. (1977) 'Social Control and the Prevention of Riots in England 1789–1829', in A.P. Donajgrodski (ed.) *Social Control in Nineteenth Century Britain*, London: Croom Helm.

Stinson, S. and Kerr, J. (eds) (1986) *International Issues in Nursing Research*, London: Croom Helm.

Stocks, M. (1960) *A Hundred Years of District Nursing*, London: Allen and Unwin.

Storch, R. (1977) 'The Problem of Working-Class Leisure — some roots of middle-class moral reform in the Industrial North 1825–50', in A.P. Donajgrodski (ed.) *Social Control in Nineteenth Century Britain*, London: Croom Helm.

Strong, P.M (1979) *The Ceremonial Order of the Clinic*, London: Routledge & Kegan Paul.

Strong, P.M. (1988) 'Minor Courtesies and Macro Structures', in P. Drew and A.J. Wootton (eds) *Erving Goffman and the Interaction Order*, Cambridge, UK: Polity Press.

Strong, P.M. and Davis, A.G. (1977) 'Roles, Role Formats and Medical Encounters: A Cross-Cultural Analysis of Staff-Client Relationships in Children's Clinics', *Sociological Review* 25: 775–800.

Sturges, O. (1880) 'Doctors and Nurses', *The Nineteenth Century* 40: 1089–96.

Summers, A. (1979) 'A Home from Home – Women's Philanthropic Work in the Nineteenth Century', in S. Burman (ed.) *Fit Work for Women*, London: Croom Helm.

Summers, A. (1983) 'Pride and Prejudice: Ladies and Nurses in the Crimean War', *History Workshop* 16: 33–56.

Summers, A. (1988) *Angels and Citizens: British Women as Military Nurses 1854–1914*, London: Routledge & Kegan Paul.

Supple, B. (1974) 'Legislation and Virtue: An Essay on Working-Class Self-Help and the State in the Early Nineteenth Century', in N. McKendrick (ed.) *Historical Perspectives: Studies in English Thought and Society in Honour of J.H. Plumb*, London: Europe Publications.

Swinburne, D. (1941) *Hospital Nurse*, London: Herbert Jenkins.

Thane, P. (1981) 'Childhood in History', in M. King (ed.) *Childhood, Welfare and Justice*, London: Batsford.

Thompson, E.P. (1967) 'Time, Work Discipline and Industrial Capitalism', *Past and Present* 38: 56–97.

Thompson, E.P. (1968) *The Making of the English Working Class*, Harmondsworth: Penguin.

Titmuss, R.M. (1958) *Essays on the Welfare State*, London: Allen and Unwin.

Tooley, S. (1906) *The History of Nursing in the British Empire*, London: Bousfield.

Towell, D. and Harries, C. (eds) (1979) *Innovation in Patient Care*, London: Croom Helm.

Towler, J. and Bramall, J. (1986) *Midwives in History and Society*, London: Croom Helm.

Turner, B. (1978) *Man-Made Disasters*, London: Taylor and Francis.

Turner, C. and Hodge, M.N. (1970) 'Occupations and Professions', in J.A. Jackson (ed.) *Professions and Professionalisation*, Cambridge, UK: Cambridge University Press.

United Kingdom Central Council for Nursing, Midwifery and Health Visiting (1986), *Project 2000: A New Preparation for Practice*, London: UKCC.

United Kingdom Central Council for Nursing, Midwifery and Health Visiting (1987) *Project 2000: The Final Proposals*, Project Paper 9, UKCC, London.

Unsworth, C. (1987) *The Politics of Mental Health Legislation*, Oxford, Clarendon Press.

Waddington, I. (1973) 'The Role of the Hospital in the Development of Modern Medicine: A Sociological Analysis', *Sociology* 7: 211–24.

Waddington, I. (1985) *The Medical Profession in the Industrial Revolution*, Dublin: Gill and Macmillan.

Walk, A. (1961) 'The History of Mental Nursing', *Journal of Mental Science* 107: 1–17.

Walton, J. (1981) 'The Treatment of Pauper Lunatics in Victorian England: the Case of the Lancaster Asylum, 1866–70', in A. Scull (ed.) *Madhouses, Mad-Doctors and Madmen*, London: Athlone.

Weber, M. (1947) *The Theory of Social and Economic Organisation*, New York: Free Press.

Webster, C. (1985) 'Nursing and the Crisis of the Early National Health Service', *Bulletin of the History of Nursing Group* 7: 4–12.

Webster, C. (1988) *Problems of Health Care: The British National Health Service Before 1957*, London: HMSO.

References

White, R. (1976) 'Some Political Influences Surrounding the Nurses' Registration Act', *Journal of Advanced Nursing*: 209–17.

White, R. (1978) *Social Change and the Development of the Nursing Profession: A Study of the Poor Law Nursing Service 1848–1948*, London: Henry Kimpton.

White, R. (1982) 'The Effects of the NHS on the Nursing Profession 1948–1961', unpublished Ph.D. thesis, University of Manchester.

White, R. (1985) *The Effects of the NHS on the Nursing Profession 1948–1961*, London: Kings Fund.

Whittaker, E.W. and Oleson, V.L. (1964) 'The Faces of Florence Nightingale: Functions of the Heroine Legend in an Occupational Sub-culture', *Human Organization* 23: 123–30.

Wilensky, H. (1964) 'The Professionalization of Everyone?', *American Journal of Sociology* 70:142–6.

Williams, K. (1980) 'From Sarah Gamp to Florence Nightingale: A Critical Survey of Hospital Nursing Systems from 1840 to 1897', in C. Davies (ed.) *Rewriting Nursing History*, London: Croom Helm.

Winter, J.M. (1977) 'The Impact of the First World War on Civilian Health in Britain', *Economic History Review* 30: 487–507.

Winter, J.M. (1979) 'Infant Mortality, Maternal Mortality and Public Health in Britain during the 1930s', *Journal of European Economic History* 8: 439–62.

Winter, J.M. (1982) 'The Decline of Mortality in Britain 1870–1950', in T. Barker and M. Drake (eds) *Population and Society in Britain 1850–1950*, London: Batsford.

Woodham-Smith, C. (1950) *Florence Nightingale*, London: Constable.

Woodward, J. (1974) *To Do the Sick No Harm: A Study of the British Voluntary Hospital System to 1875*, London: Routledge & Kegan Paul.

Wrigley, E.A. (1969) *Population and History*, London: Weidenfeld and Nicolson.

Yeo, S. (1979) 'Working Class Association, Private Capital, Welfare and the State in the Late Nineteenth and Early Twentieth Centuries', in N. Parry, M. Rustin and C. Satyamurti (eds) *Social Work, Welfare and the State*, London: Edward Arnold.

250

Index

Index